CLINICAL HEMATOLOGY ATLAS

CLINICAL HEMATOLOGY ATLAS

Jacqueline H. Carr, MS, MT(ASCP)SH, DLM

Department of Pathology and Laboratory Medicine
Division of Hematopathology
Indiana University Medical Center
Indianapolis, Indiana

Bernadette F. Rodak, MS, CLSpH(NCA), MT(ASCP)SH

Associate Professor
Medical Technology Program
School for Allied Health Sciences
Indiana University
Indianapolis, Indiana

W.B. SAUNDERS COMPANY
A Division of Harcourt Brace & Company

Philadelphia   London   Toronto   Montreal   Sydney   Tokyo

W.B. SAUNDERS COMPANY
A Division of Harcourt Brace & Company

The Curtis Center
Independence Square West
Philadelphia, Pennsylvania 19106

Library of Congress Cataloging-In-Publication Data

Carr, Jacqueline H.
    Clinical hematology atlas / Jacqueline H. Carr, Bernadette F.
Rodak.

    p.   cm.

    ISBN 0–7216–4174–1

    1. Blood—Diseases—Atlases.   2. Hematology—Atlases.   I. Rodak,
    Bernadette F.   II. Title.
    [DNLM: 1. Hematologic Diseases—diagnosis atlases.   2. Hematologic
    Diseases—pathology atlases.   WH 17 C311c 1999]
    RB145.C26   1999   616. 1'5'00222—dc21

    DNLM/DLC   98-5824

CLINICAL HEMATOLOGY ATLAS   ISBN 0–7216–4174–1

Printed in the United States of America.

Last digit is the print number: 9   8   7   6   5   4   3   2

PREFACE

Although there are several excellent hematology atlases available for use on personal computers and on the Internet, in most instances this electronic medium does not lend itself well to morphologists who benefit by having photographs available when cells must be identified. Since the emphasis of an atlas is morphology, the *Clinical Hematology Atlas* is intended to be used with a textbook, such as *Diagnostic Hematology* by Rodak, that addresses physiology and diagnosis, along with morphology.

This atlas is designed for a diverse audience that includes clinical laboratory science students, medical students, residents, and practitioners. It will also be a valuable resource for clinical laboratory practitioners who are being retrained or cross-trained in hematology.

As is frequently expounded, "morphology on a peripheral blood film is only as good as the quality of the smear and the stain." Chapter 1 reviews smear preparation, staining, and the appropriate area in which to evaluate cell distribution and morphology.

Chapter 2 schematically presents hematopoietic features of cell maturation. General cell maturation, along with an electron micrograph with labeled organelles, will help the user correlate the sub-structures with the appearance of cells under light microscopy. Visualizing *normal* cellular maturation is essential to the understanding of disease processes. This correlation of schematic, electron micrograph, and Wright stained morphology is carried throughout the maturation chapters.

Chapters 3 to 9 present the maturation of each cell line individually, repeating the respective segment of the overall hematopoietic scheme from Chapter 2 in order to assist the student in seeing the relationship of each cell line to the whole. In these chapters, each maturation stage is presented as a color print, a schematic, and an electron micrograph. A description of each cell, including overall size, nuclear to cytoplasmic ratio, morphologic features, and reference ranges in peripheral blood and bone marrow serve as a convenient summary. The final figure in each of these chapters summarizes lineage maturation by repeating the hematopoietic segment, with the corresponding photomicrographs.

Chapters 10 to 12 present discrete cellular abnormalities of erythrocytes, that is, variations in size, color, shape, and distribution, as well as inclusions found in erythrocytes. Each variation is presented along with a description of the abnormality, or composition of the inclusion, and associated disorders.

Since diseases are often combinations of the cellular alterations, Chapter 13 integrates morphologic findings into the diagnostic features of disorders primarily affecting erythrocytes.

In Chapters 14 and 15, nuclear and cytoplasmic alterations of leukocytes are displayed as a stepping stone to the correlations with leukocyte disorders.

Diseases of excessive or altered production of cells may be due to maturation arrest, asynchronous development, or proliferation of one cell line, as presented in Chapters 15 to 20.

It is the design of the authors that the cellular defects in leukocyte disorders be visually compared with the process of normal hematopoiesis for a more thorough comprehension of normal and altered development. The reader is encouraged to refer to the normal hematopoiesis illustration, Figure 2-1, for comparison of normal and abnormal cells and the progression of diseases.

Chapter 21 presents the most common stains, along with a summary chart for interpretation. Cytochemical stains aid in the diagnosis of leukoproliferative disorders.

Microorganisms, including parasites, may be seen on peripheral blood smears. A brief photographic overview is given in Chapter 22. The reader is encouraged to consult a microbiology reference, such as *Textbook of Diagnostic Microbiology* by Connie Mahon and George Manuselis, for a more detailed presentation.

Chapter 23 includes photomicrographs that are not categorized into any one particular area, such as fat cells, mitotic figures, metastatic tumor cells, and artifact.

All of these chapters combine into what we feel is a comprehensive and valuable resource for any clinical laboratory. The quality of the schematic illustrations, electron micrographs, and color photographs stand for themselves. We hope that this atlas will enrich the learning process for the student and serve as an important reference tool for the practitioner.

Jacqueline Hart Carr

Bernadette F. Rodak

ACKNOWLEDGMENTS

From inception to completion we have had a great deal of assistance and encouragement from the faculty and staff of the Indiana University School of Allied Health Sciences and the Department of Pathology and Laboratory Medicine, Indiana University Medical Center. The following individuals have "gone the extra mile" to help us realize our "dream." **Carol Bradford,** MT(ASCP)SH, Department of Medicine; for putting her extensive slide collection at our disposal; **George Girgis,** MT(ASCP), for his perseverance in locating specimens and his willingness to coverslip an incredible number of slides; **Michael Goheen,** MS, Supervisor of the Electron Microscopy Laboratory, for his expertise and patience; **John Griep,** MD, Clinical Professor of Pathology, Indiana University, and Medical Director of Pathology and Laboratory Service, St. Catherine Hospital, East Chicago, IL, for his expert advice and moral support; **Saeed Kahn,** DVM, who patiently prepared samples for electron microscopy; **Nancy Maguire,** for her cheerfulness and gracious acceptance of the extra work this book added to her film processing responsibilities; **Richard Neiman,** MD, Director, Division of Hematopathology, for support; **Gary Schmitt,** graphic artist in the Medical Illustrations Department, who sees color a lot more clearly than we do; **Marcella Liffick Stevens,** MA, MS, CLS(NCA), MT(ASCP), who shared her ideas and concepts with us in the embryonic stages of this atlas.

A special thank you to the professionals at the W.B. Saunders Company, who navigated us through the production of this atlas. **Rachael Kelly,** Developmental Editor, who persevered with us and encouraged us through some rough times; **Selma Kaszczuk,** former Senior Acquisitions Editor, and **Adrienne Williams,** Acquisitions Editor; **Agnes Byrne,** Project Editor; **Denise LeMelledo,** Production Manager; and **Lisa Lambert,** Illustration Coordinator.

Jacqueline Hart Carr

Bernadette F. Rodak

CONTENTS

1

Introduction to Peripheral Blood Smear Examination

A properly prepared blood smear is essential to accurate assessment of cellular morphology. A variety of methods are available for preparing and staining blood smears, the most common of which are discussed here. It is beyond the scope of this atlas to discuss other methodologies; however, detailed descriptions of these procedures can be found in a textbook of hematology.

■ WEDGE SMEAR PREPARATION

The wedge smear is the most convenient and commonly used technique for making peripheral blood smears. This technique requires at least two 3 × 1 inch (75 × 25 mm) clean glass slides. High-quality, beveled-edge microscope slides are recommended. One slide serves as the blood smear slide and the other as the spreader slide; these can then be reversed to prepare a second smear. A drop of ethylenediaminetetra-acetic acid (EDTA) anticoagulated blood about 3 mm in diameter is placed at one end of the slide. Alternatively, a similar size drop of blood directly from a finger or heel puncture is acceptable. The size of the drop of blood is important: too large a drop creates very long or thick smears and too small a drop often makes a short or thin smear. In preparing the smear, the pusher slide is held securely in front of the drop of blood at a 30- to 45-degree angle to the smear slide (Fig. 1–1A). The pusher slide is pulled back into the drop of blood and held in that position until the blood spreads across the width of the slide (Fig. 1–1B). It is then quickly and smoothly pushed forward to the end of the smear slide, creating a wedge smear (Fig. 1–1C). It is important that the whole drop of blood is picked up and spread. Moving the pusher slide forward too slowly accentuates poor leukocyte distribution by pushing larger cells, such as monocytes and granulocytes, to the very end and sides of the smear. Maintaining a consistent angle between the slides and an even, gentle pressure is essential. It is frequently necessary to adjust the angle between the slides to produce a satisfactory smear. For higher-than-normal hematocrit, the angle between the slides must be lowered so that the smear is not too short and thick. For extremely low hematocrit, the angle must be raised. A well-made peripheral blood smear (Fig. 1–2) has the following characteristics:

1. About two thirds to three fourths of the length of the slide is covered by the smear.

2. It is very slightly rounded at feather edge (thin portion), not bullet-shaped.

3. Lateral edges of the smear should be visible. The use of slides with chamfered (beveled) corners may facilitate this appearance.

4. It is smooth without irregularities, holes, or streaks.

5. When the slide is held up to light, the feather edge of the smear should have a "rainbow" appearance.

6. The whole drop is picked up and spread.

Figure 1–3 shows examples of unacceptable smears.

Staining of Peripheral Blood Smears

The purpose of staining blood smears is to identify cells and recognize morphology easily through the microscope. Wright stain or Wright-Giemsa stain is the most commonly used stain for peripheral blood and bone marrow smears. These contain both eosin and methylene blue and are therefore termed polychrome stains.

The cells are fixed to the glass slide by the methanol in the stain. Staining reactions are pH dependent, and the actual staining of the cellular components occurs when a buffer (pH 6.4) is added to the stain. Free methylene blue is basic and stains acidic cellular compo-

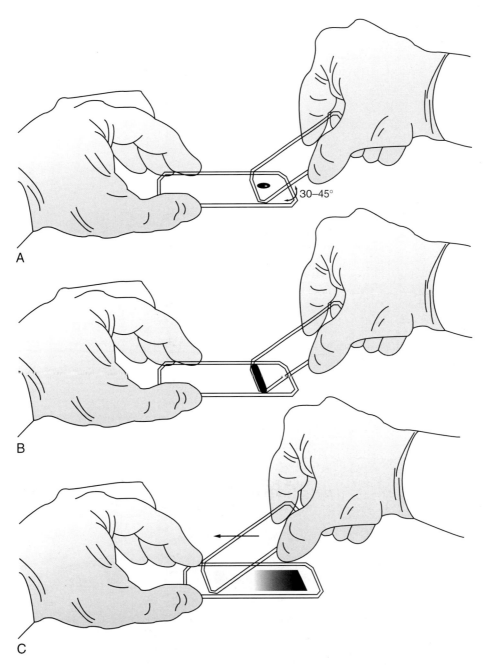

Figure 1–1 Wedge technique of making a peripheral blood smear. **A,** Correct angle to hold spreader slide. **B,** Blood spread across width of slide. **C,** Completed wedge smear. (From Rodak BF: Diagnostic Hematology. Philadelphia, WB Saunders, 1995.)

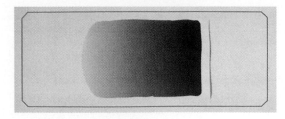

Figure 1–2 Well-made peripheral blood smear. (From Rodak BF: Diagnostic Hematology. Philadelphia, WB Saunders, 1995.)

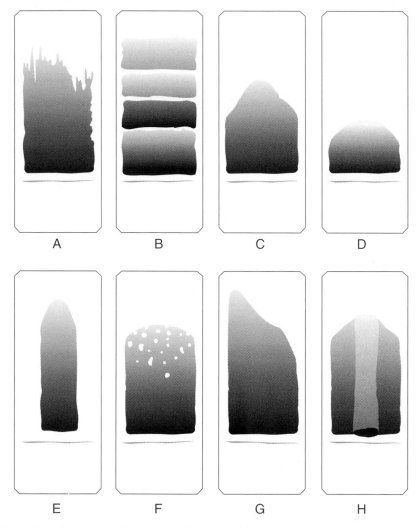

Figure 1–3 Examples of unacceptable smears. (From Rodak BF: Diagnostic Hematology. Philadelphia, WB Saunders, 1995.)

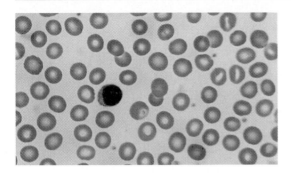

Figure 1–4   Optimally stained peripheral blood smear demonstrating the appropriate area in which to perform the WBC differential and morphology assessment and the platelet estimate. Only the center of the field is shown; an entire field would contain 200 to 250 RBCs (×1000).

nents, such as RNA, blue. Free eosin is acidic and stains basic components, such as hemoglobin or eosinophilic granules, red. Neutrophils have cytoplasmic granules that have a neutral pH and accept some characteristics from both stains. Details for specific methods of staining peripheral and bone marrow smears may be found in a standard textbook of hematology.

An optimally stained smear (Fig. 1–4) has the following characteristics:

1. The red blood cells (RBCs) should be pink to salmon in color.

2. Nuclei are dark blue to purple.

3. Cytoplasmic granules of neutrophils are lilac.

4. Cytoplasmic granules of basophils are dark blue to black.

5. Cytoplasmic granules of eosinophils are red to orange.

6. The area between the cells should be clean and free of precipitated stain.

A well-stained slide is necessary for accurate interpretation of cellular morphology. The best staining results are obtained from freshly made slides that have been prepared within 2 to 3 hours of blood collection. Slides must be allowed to dry throughly before staining. Table 1–1 lists common reasons for poorly stained slides and may be used as a guide when troubleshooting.

■ PERIPHERAL SMEAR EXAMINATION

Examination of the blood smear is a multistep process. The smear examination begins with a scan of the slide at 10× or low power. This step is necessary to assess the overall quality of the smear, including abnormal distribution of RBCs suggesting the presence of rouleaux or autoagglutination and/or the presence of a disproportionate number of large nucleated cells such as monocytes or neutrophils at the edges of the smear. If the latter exists, another smear

Table 1–1   TROUBLESHOOTING POORLY STAINED BLOOD SMEARS

First Scenario
Problems
Red blood cells appear gray
White blood cells are too dark
Eosinophil granules are gray, not orange

Causes
Stain or buffer too alkaline (most common)
Inadequate rinsing
Prolonged staining

Second Scenario
Problems
Red blood cells too pale or red color
White blood cells barely visible

Causes
Stain or buffer too acidic (most common)
Underbuffering (too short)
Overrinsing

From Rodak BF: Diagnostic Hematology. Philadelphia, WB Saunders, 1995.

should be prepared. Additionally, the 10× smear examination allows for the rapid detection of large abnormal cells such as blasts, reactive lymphocytes, and parasites.

Using the 40× (high dry) objective, find an area of the smear in which the RBCs are evenly distributed and barely touching one another (two or three cells may overlap) (Fig. 1–5). Eight to 10 fields in this area of the smear are scanned and the average number of

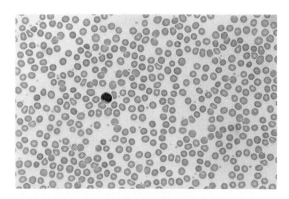

Figure 1–5   Correct area of blood smear in which to evaluate cellular distribution and perform WBC estimate (×400).

white blood cells (WBCs) per field is determined. The average number of WBCs per high power field is multiplied by 2000 to get an approximation of the total WBC count/mm^3. This estimate is a useful quality control tool for validating WBC counts from hematology analyzers. Any discrepancy between the instrument WBC count and the slide estimate must be resolved. Some reasons for discrepancy are mislabeled smear, smear made from the wrong patient's sample, and instrument malfunction.

The next step in smear evaluation is to perform the WBC differential. This is done in the same area of the smear as the WBC estimate, but using the 100× oil immersion objective. When the correct area of a specimen from a patient with a normal RBC count is viewed, about 200 to 250 RBCs per oil immersion field are seen (see Fig. 1–4). Characteristically, the differential count includes counting and classifying 100 WBCs and reporting these classes as percentages. The RBC, WBC, and platelet morphology evaluations and the platelet estimates are also performed under the 100× oil immersion objective. RBC inclusions, such as Howell-Jolly bodies, and white blood cell inclusions, like Döhle bodies, can be seen at this magnification. When present, nucleated red blood cells (NRBCs) are counted and reported as number of NRBCs/100 WBCs. The differential count is performed in a systematic manner using a "battlement" track (Fig. 1–6), which minimizes WBC distribution errors. One hundred consecutive WBCs are counted and classified. The results are reported as percentages of each type of WBC seen during the count. An example of a WBC differential count is 3% bands, 55% polymorphonuclear neutrophils, 30% lymphocytes, 6% monocytes, 4% eosinophils, and 2% basophils. Any WBC abnormalities such as toxic changes, Döhle bodies, reactive lymphocytes, and Auer rods are also reported. Each laboratory should have established protocols for the standardized reporting of abnormalities.

Evaluation of the RBC morphology is an important aspect of the smear evaluation and is used in conjunction with the RBC indices to describe cells as normal or abnormal in size, shape, and color. Most laboratories use concise statements describing overall RBC morphology that is consistent with the RBC indices. The micro-

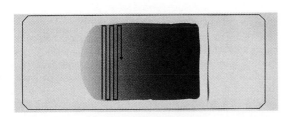

Figure 1–6 "Battlement" pattern for performing a WBC differential. (From Rodak BF: Diagnostic Hematology. Philadelphia, WB Saunders, 1995.)

scopic evaluation of RBC morphology must be congruent with the information given by the automated hematology analyzer. If not, discrepancies must be resolved before reporting patient results.

The final step in the performance of the differential count is the estimation of the platelet number. This is done under the 100× oil immersion objective. In an area of the smear where RBCs barely touch, the number of platelets in 10 oil immersion fields is counted. The average number of platelets is multiplied by 20,000 to provide an estimation of the total number of platelets present in the sample. This estimate is reported as adequate if the estimate is consistent with a normal platelet count, decreased if below the lower limit of normal for that laboratory, and increased if above the upper limit of normal. (A general reference range is 150 to 450 $\times$ 10^9/L). The estimate can be compared with an automated platelet count as an additional quality control measure.

It should be noted that high-quality, 40× or 50× oil immersion objectives can be used by the experienced technologist to perform the differential analysis of the blood smear. However, all abnormal findings must be verified under the 100× objective.

◼ SUMMARY

A considerable amount of valuable information can be obtained from properly prepared, stained, and examined peripheral blood smears. Most laboratories use smears made by the wedge technique from EDTA anticoagulated blood and stained with Wright or Wright-Giemsa stain. The smears should be evaluated in a systematic manner using first the 10×, then 40× high dry, and finally the 100× oil immersion objectives on the microscope. White blood cell differential and morphology, as well as the RBC morphology and platelet estimate, are included in the smear evaluation.

CHAPTER

2

Hematopoiesis

Hematopoiesis is a vigorous process of blood cell production and maturation that occurs primarily in the bone marrow. The process begins with the pluripotential stem cell that is capable of proliferation, replication, and differentiation. In response to cytokines (growth factors), the pluripotential stem cell will differentiate into a myeloid or a lymphoid stem cell. Both the myeloid and lymphoid stem cells maintain their pluripotential capacity. The lymphoid stem cell differentiates into a committed pre-B or pre-T stem cell. The myeloid stem cell produces an intermediate stem cell, CFU–GEMM (colony forming unit–granulocyte, erythrocyte, monocyte, megakaryocyte), which, in response to specific cytokines, differentiates into erythroid, megakaryocytic, myeloid, monocytic, eosinophilic, or basophilic lineage. To this point in maturation, none of these stem cells may be morphologically identified, although it is postulated that they appear similar to a small resting lymphocyte. The shaded area in Figure 2–1 highlights the stem cell populations. Each lineage and maturation stage will be presented in detail in the following chapters.

Hematopoiesis is a dynamic continuum, that is, cells gradually mature from one stage to the next and may be between stages when viewed through the microscope. In general, the cell is then identified as the more mature stage. Figures 2–2 and 2–3 illustrate cell ultrastructure. Review of organelles will facilitate correlation of morphologic maturation with cell function. This topic is explored in depth in hematology textbooks. Table 2–1 delineates the location, appearance, and function of individual organelles. General morphologic changes in blood cell maturation (Fig. 2–4) include

- Basophilic cytoplasm to less basophilic
- Reduction in cell size
- Condensation of nuclear chromatin

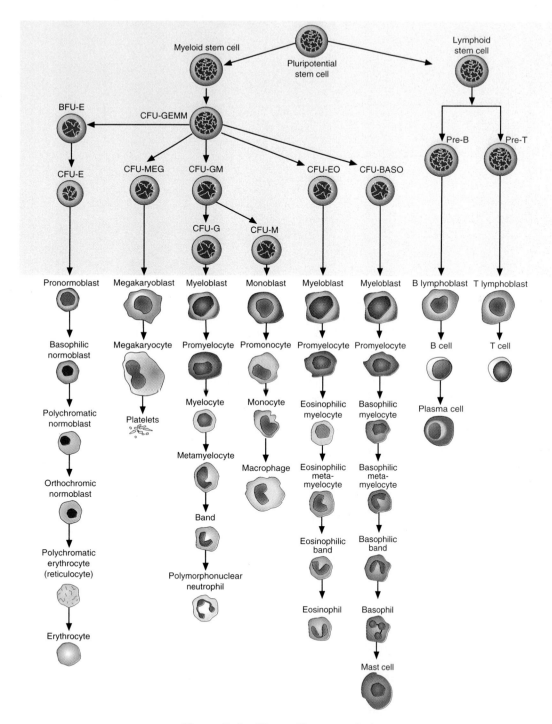

Figure 2–1 Chart of hematopoiesis.

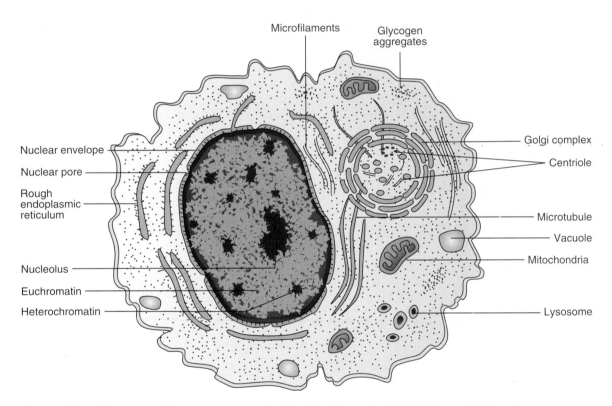

Figure 2–2   Schematic of electron micrograph. (Modified from Rodak BF: Diagnostic Hematology. Philadelphia, WB Saunders, 1995.)

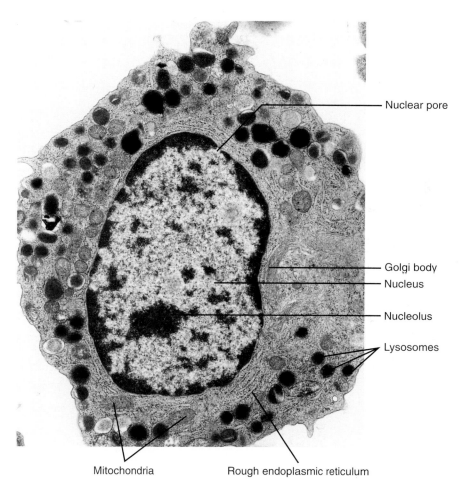

Nuclear pore

Golgi body

Nucleus

Nucleolus

Lysosomes

Mitochondria

Rough endoplasmic reticulum

Figure 2–3 Electron micrograph with labeled organelles.

Table 2–1 SUMMARY OF CELLULAR COMPONENTS AND FUNCTIONS

Organelle	Location	Appearance and Size	Function	Comments
Membranes: plasma, nuclear, mitochondrial, endoplasmic reticulum	Outer boundary of cell, nucleus, endoplasmic reticulum, mitochondria and other organelles	Usually a lipid bilayer consisting of proteins, cholesterol, phospholipids, and polysaccharides; membrane thickness varies with the cell or organelle	Separates the various cellular components; facilitates and restricts cellular exchange of substances	Membrane must be resilient and flexible
Nucleus	Within cell	Usually round or oval but varies depending on cell; varies in size; composed of DNA	The control center of the cell and contains the genetic blueprint	Governs the cellular activity and transmits information for cellular control
Nucleolus	Within nucleus	Usually round or irregular in shape; 2–4 μ in size; composed of RNA; there may be 1–4 within nucleus	Site of synthesis and processing of various ribosomal RNA	Appearance varies with activity of the cells; larger when cell is actively involved in protein synthesis
Golgi body	Between nucleus and luminal surface of the cell	System of stacked membrane-bound flattened sacs; varies in size	Involved in modifying and packaging macromolecules for secretion	Well developed in cells with large secretion responsibilities
Endoplasmic reticulum	Randomly throughout cytoplasm	Membrane-lined tubules that branch and connect to nucleus and plasma membrane	Stores and transports fluids and chemicals	Two types: smooth with no ribosomes; rough with ribosomes on the surface

	Location	Structure	Function	Comments
Ribosomes	Free in cytoplasm. Outer surface of rough endoplasmic reticulum	Small granule, 100–300 Å; composed of protein and nucleic acid	Protein production, such as enzymes and blood proteins	Large proteins are synthesized from polyribosomes (chains of ribosomes)
Mitochondria	Randomly in cytoplasm	Round or oval structures; 3–14 nm in length, 2–10 nm in width; membrane has 2 layers; inner layer has folds called cristae	Cell's "powerhouse"; makes ATP, the energy source for the cell	Active cells have more present than do inactive ones
Lysosomes	Randomly in cytoplasm	Membrane bound sacs; size varies	Contain hydrolytic enzymes for cellular digestive system	If the membrane breaks, the hydrolytic enzymes can destroy the cell
Microfilaments	Near nuclear envelope and within proximity of mitotic process	Small, solid structure approximately 5 nm in diameter	Support of cytoskeleton and motility	Consist of actin and myosin (contractile proteins)
Microtubules	Cytoskeleton, near nuclear envelope and component part of centriole near Golgi body	Hollow cylinder with protofilaments surrounding the outside tube; 20–25 nm in diameter, variable length	Maintenance of cell shape, motility, and the mitotic process	Produced from tubulin polymerization; make up mitotic spindles and part of the structure of centriole.
Centriole	In centrosome near nucleus	Cylinders; 150 nm in diameter, 300–500 nm in length	Serve as insertion points for mitotic spindle fibers	Nine sets of triplet microtubules

From Rodak BF: Diagnostic Hematology. Philadelphia, WB Saunders, 1995.

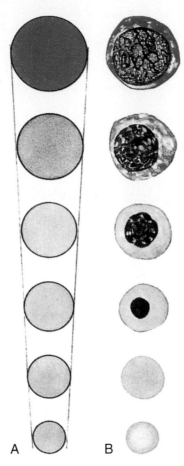

A   B

Figure 2–4 A,   General cellular maturation: Changes in cell size and color.   **B,**   General cell maturation: Changes in nuclear size and chromatin condensation. Note: Red blood cell loses nucleus. White blood cell nucleus is retained and undergoes further maturation. (From Diggs LW, Sturm D, and Bell A: The Morphology of Human Blood Cells, 5th ed. Abbott Park, IL, Abbott Laboratories, 1985. Reproduction of *Morphology of Human Blood Cells* has been granted with approval of Abbott Laboratories, all rights reserved by Abbott Laboratories.)

3

Erythroid Maturation

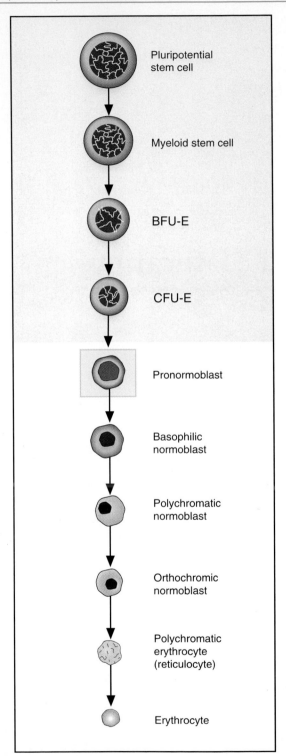

Figure 3–1   Erythroid sequence—Pronormoblast

PRONORMOBLAST

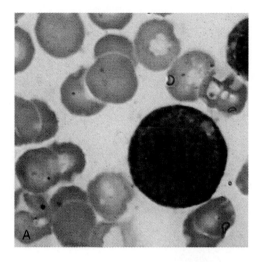

Figure 3–2A   Pronormoblast

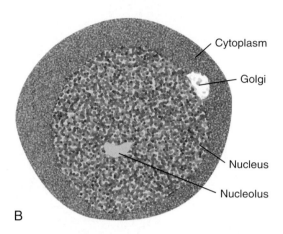

Figure 3–2B   Schematic of pronormoblast

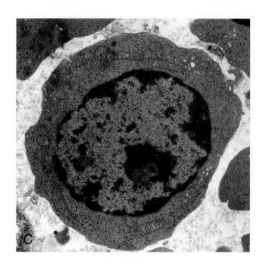

Figure 3–2C   Electron micrograph of
pronormoblast (×15,575)

SIZE: 12–20μ
NUCLEUS: Round
    Nucleoli: 1–2
    Chromatin: Fine
CYTOPLASM: Dark blue

N/C RATIO: 8:1
REFERENCE INTERVAL:
    Bone Marrow: 1%
    Peripheral Blood: 0%

All photomicrographs are ×1000 with Wright-Giemsa stain unless stated otherwise.

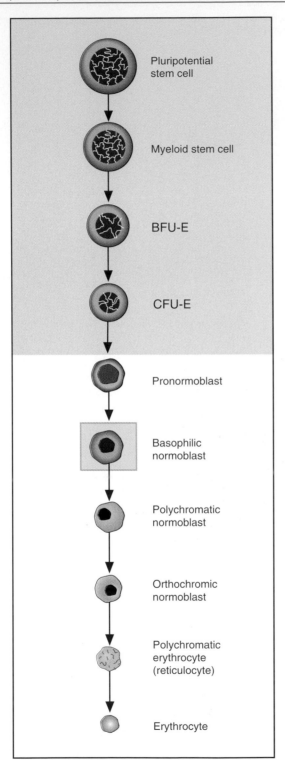

Figure 3–3   Erythroid sequence—Basophilic normoblast

BASOPHILIC NORMOBLAST

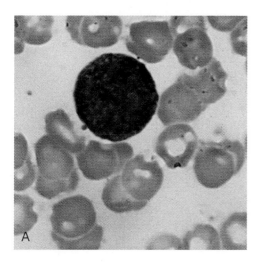

Figure 3–4A Basophilic normoblast

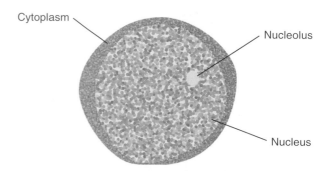

Figure 3–4B Schematic of basophilic normoblast

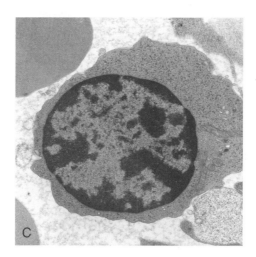

Figure 3–4C Electron micrograph of
basophilic normoblast (×15,575)

SIZE: 10–15μ
NUCLEUS: Round
  Nucleoli: 0–1
  Chromatin: Slightly condensed
CYTOPLASM: Dark blue

N/C RATIO: 6:1
REFERENCE INTERVAL:
 Bone Marrow: 1–4%
 Peripheral Blood: 0%

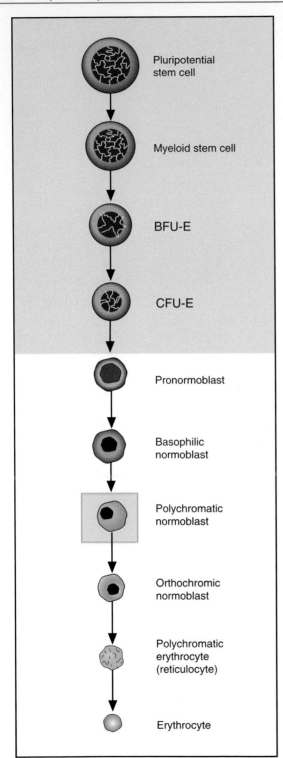

Figure 3–5 Erythroid sequence—Polychromatic normoblast

POLYCHROMATIC NORMOBLAST

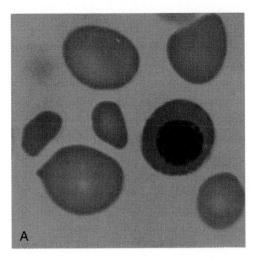

Figure 3–6A   Polychromatic normoblast

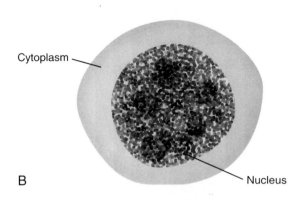

Figure 3–6B   Schematic of polychromatic normoblast

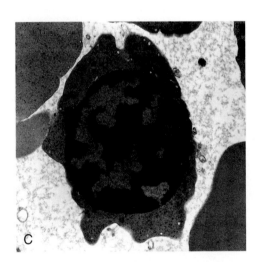

Figure 3–6C   Electron micrograph of
polychromatic normoblast (×15,575)

SIZE: 10–12μ
NUCLEUS: Round
    Nucleoli: 0
    Chromatin: Quite condensed
CYTOPLASM: Gray blue

N/C RATIO: 4:1
REFERENCE INTERVAL:
    Bone Marrow: 10–20%
    Peripheral Blood: 0%

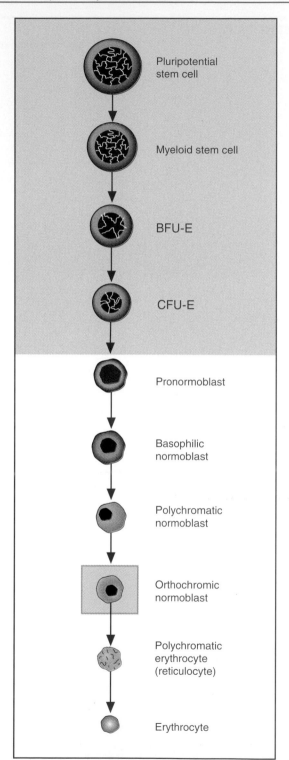

Pluripotential stem cell

Myeloid stem cell

BFU-E

CFU-E

Pronormoblast

Basophilic normoblast

Polychromatic normoblast

Orthochromic normoblast

Polychromatic erythrocyte (reticulocyte)

Erythrocyte

Figure 3–7 Erythroid sequence—Orthochromic normoblast

ORTHOCHROMATIC NORMOBLAST

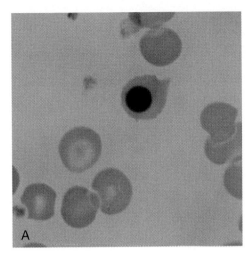

Figure 3–8A Orthochromic normoblast

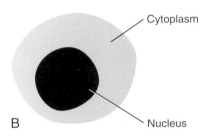

B

Figure 3–8B Schematic of orthochromic normoblast

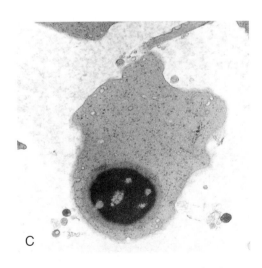

C

Figure 3–8C Electron micrograph of orthochromic normoblast (×20,125)

SIZE: 8–10μ
NUCLEUS: Round
    Nucleoli: 0
    Chromatin: Fully condensed
CYTOPLASM: Blue to salmon

N/C RATIO: 0.5:1
REFERENCE INTERVAL:
    Bone Marrow: 5–10%
    Peripheral Blood: 0%

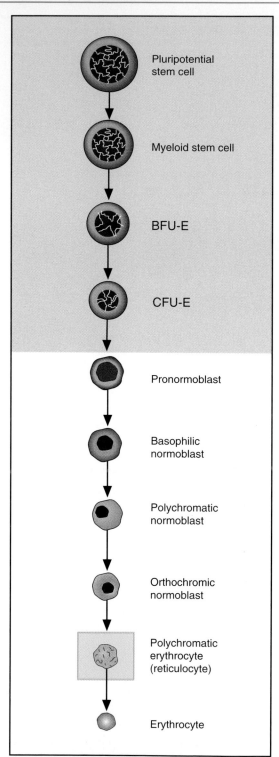

Figure 3–9 Erythroid sequence— Polychromatic erythrocyte (reticulocyte)

POLYCHROMATIC ERYTHROCYTE

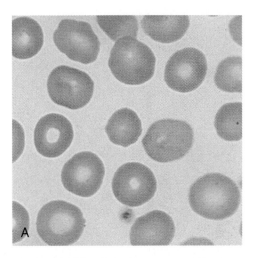

Figure 3–10A   Polychromatic erythrocyte

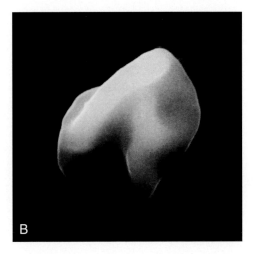

Figure 3–10B   Scanning electron micrograph of polychromatic erythrocyte (×5000)

SIZE: 8–8.5μ
NUCLEUS: Absent
   Nucleoli: NA
   Chromatin: NA
CYTOPLASM: Blue to salmon
N/C RATIO: NA

REFERENCE INTERVAL:
   Bone Marrow: 1%
   Peripheral Blood: 0.5–2.0%
NOTE: When stained with supravital stain
   (e.g., new methylene blue), polychromatic erythrocytes appear as
   reticulocytes.

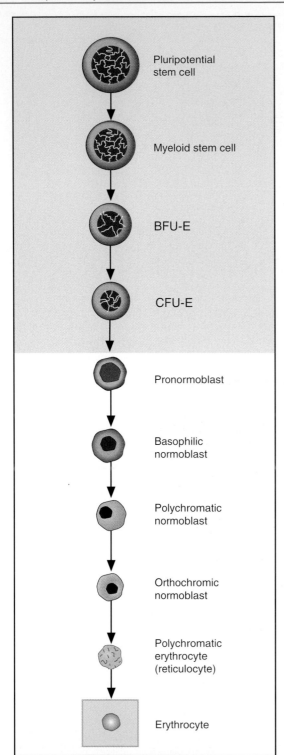

Figure 3–11 Erythroid Sequence—Erythrocyte

ERYTHROCYTE

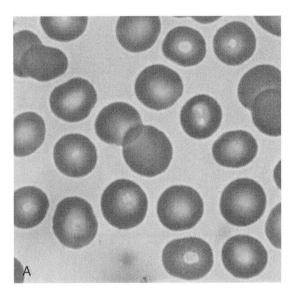

Figure 3–12A   Erythrocyte

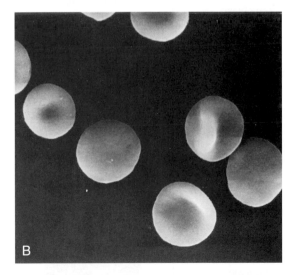

Figure 3–12B   Scanning electron micrograph of erythrocyte (×2500)

SIZE: 7–8μ

NUCLEUS: Absent

    Nucleoli: NA

    Chromatin: NA

CYTOPLASM: Salmon

N/C RATIO: NA

REFERENCE INTERVAL:

    Bone Marrow: NA

    Peripheral Blood: Predominant cell type

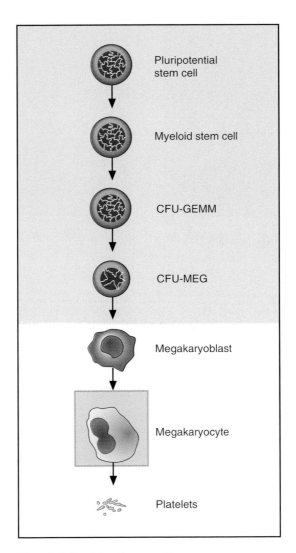

Figure 4–1 Megakaryocytic sequence—
Megakaryocyte

Megakaryoblasts cannot be identified with certainty by Wright-Giemsa stain.

MEGAKARYOCYTE

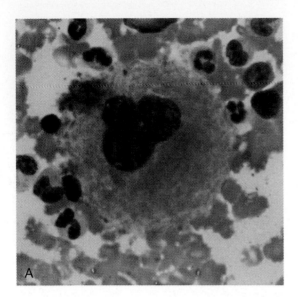

Figure 4–2A Megakaryocyte, early stage—Bone marrow (×500)

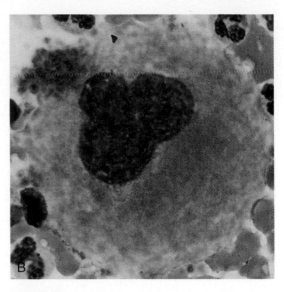

Figure 4–2B Megakaryocyte, early stage—Bone marrow (×1000)

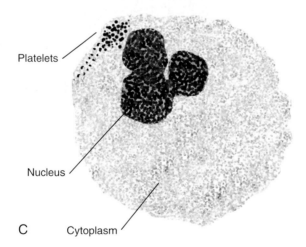

Platelets

Nucleus

C   Cytoplasm

Figure 4–2C Schematic megakaryocyte

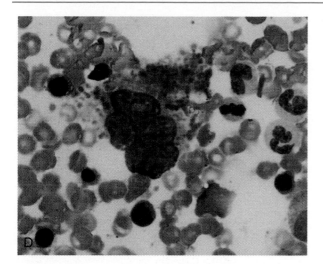

Figure 4–2D Megakaryocyte, late stage—Bone marrow (×100)

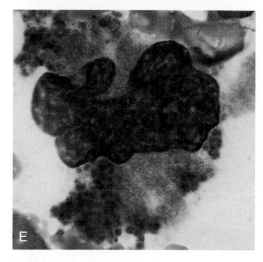

Figure 4–2E Megakaryocyte, late stage—Bone marrow (×500)

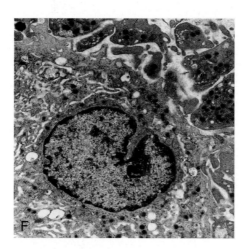

Figure 4–2F Electron micrograph of megakaryocyte (×16,500)

SIZE: 20–90μ

NUCLEUS: 2–16 lobes (8 lobes: most common)

NOTE: The size of the cell varies according to number of lobes present.

CYTOPLASM: Blue to pink; abundant

    Granules: Reddish blue; few to abundant

N/C RATIO: Variable

REFERENCE INTERVAL:

    Bone Marrow: 5–10 per 10× objective (100× magnification) 1–2 per 50× objective (500× magnification)

NOTE: Megakaryocytes are usually reported as adequate, increased, or decreased and not as a percentage.

    Peripheral Blood: 0%

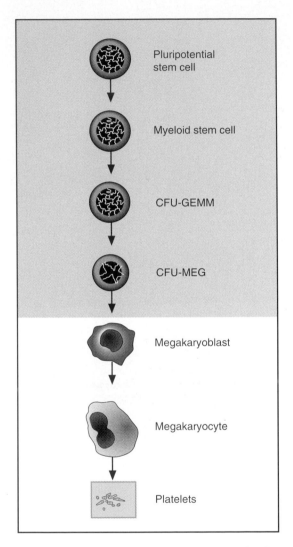

Figure 4–3   Megakaryocytic sequence—Platelets

PLATELET

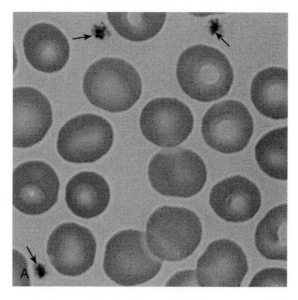

Figure 4–4A   Platelet

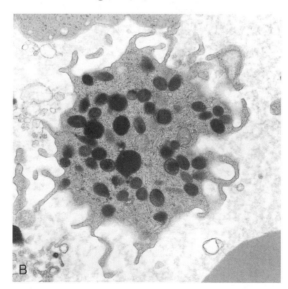

Figure 4–4B   Electron micrograph of platelet (×28,750)

SIZE: 2–4μ
NUCLEUS: NA
CYTOPLASM: Light blue to colorless
    Granules: Red to violet
N/C RATIO: NA

REFERENCE INTERVAL:
    Bone Marrow: NA
    Peripheral Blood: 7–25 per 100× oil im-
           mersion field

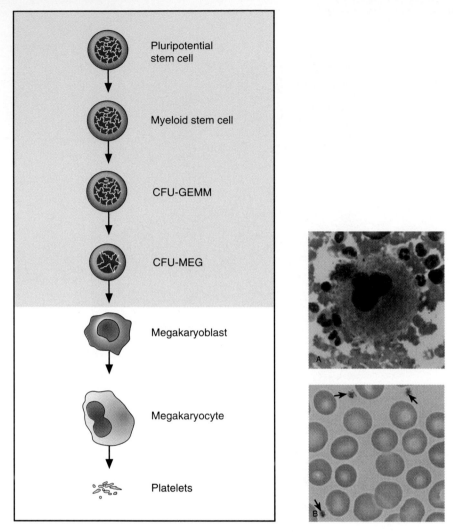

Figure 4–5 Megakaryocytic sequence with **(A)** megakaryocyte and **(B)** platelet

5

Myeloid Maturation

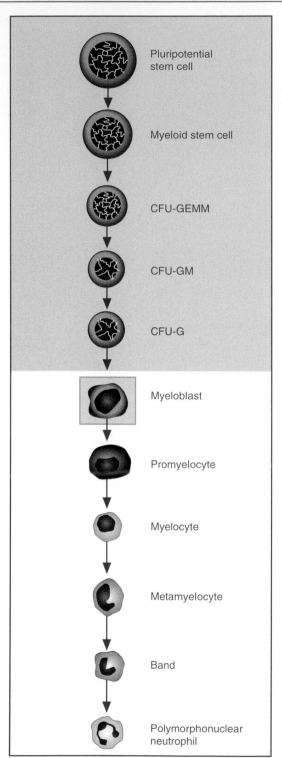

Pluripotential stem cell

Myeloid stem cell

CFU-GEMM

CFU-GM

CFU-G

Myeloblast

Promyelocyte

Myelocyte

Metamyelocyte

Band

Polymorphonuclear neutrophil

Figure 5–1 Myeloid sequence—Myeloblast

MYELOBLAST

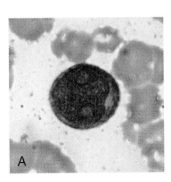

Figure 5–2A Myeloblast

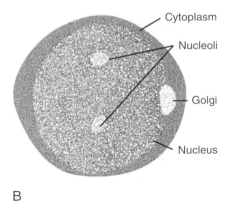

Figure 5–2B Schematic of myeloblast

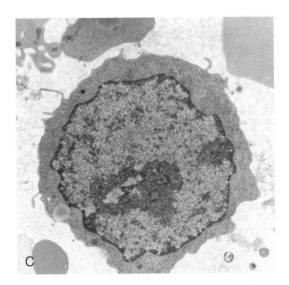

Figure 5–2C Electron micrograph of myeloblast (×16,500)

SIZE: 15–20μ
NUCLEUS: Round to oval
    Nucleoli: 2–5
    Chromatin: Fine
CYTOPLASM: Moderate basophilia
    Granules: Absent

N/C RATIO: 4:1
REFERENCE INTERVAL:
    Bone Marrow: 0–1%
    Peripheral Blood: 0%

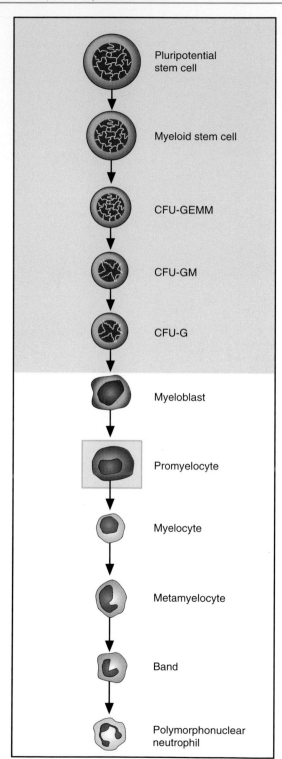

Figure 5–3   Myeloid sequence—Promyelocyte

PROMYELOCYTE

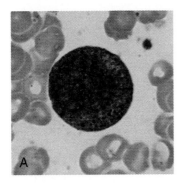

Figure 5–4A Promyelocyte

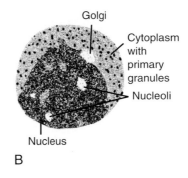

Figure 5–4B Schematic of promyelocyte

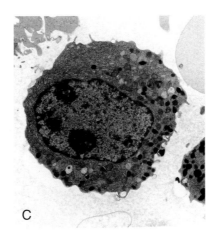

Figure 5–4C Electron micrograph of promyelocyte (×13,000)

SIZE: 14–20μ
NUCLEUS: Round to oval
      Nucleoli: 1–3 or more
      Chromatin: Slightly coarser than
            myeloblast
CYTOPLASM: Basophilic
      Granules:
            Primary: Few red to purple
            Secondary: None

N/C RATIO: 3:1
REFERENCE INTERVAL:
      Bone Marrow: 2–5%
      Peripheral Blood: 0%

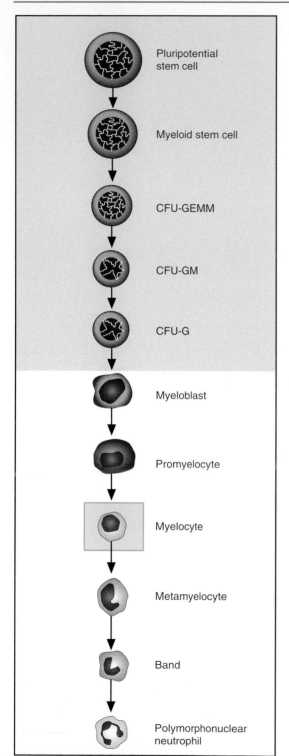

Figure 5–5 Myeloid sequence—Myelocyte

MYELOCYTE

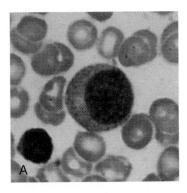

Figure 5–6A   Myelocyte

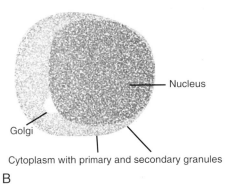

Golgi

Nucleus

Cytoplasm with primary and secondary granules

B

Figure 5–6B   Schematic of myelocyte

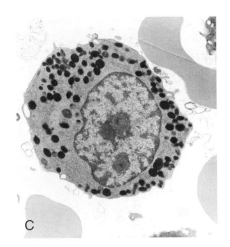

C

Figure 5–6C   Electron micrograph
of myelocyte (×16,500)

SIZE: 12–18μ
NUCLEUS: Round to oval; may have one
flattened side
Nucleoli: Usually not visible
Chromatin: Coarse and more condensed
than promyelocyte
CYTOPLASM: Slightly basophilic
Granules:
Primary: Few to moderate
Secondary: Variable number

N/C RATIO: 2:1
REFERENCE INTERVAL:
Bone Marrow: 5–19%
Peripheral Blood: 0%

(NOTE: As the cell matures, secondary granules differentiate the cell lineage into neutrophil, eosinophil, or basophil.)

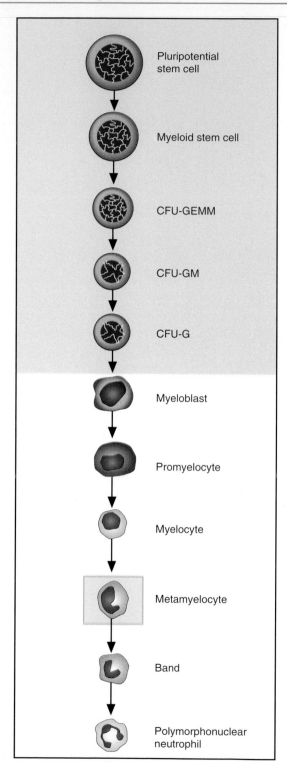

Pluripotential stem cell

Myeloid stem cell

CFU-GEMM

CFU-GM

CFU-G

Myeloblast

Promyelocyte

Myelocyte

Metamyelocyte

Band

Polymorphonuclear neutrophil

Figure 5–7   Myeloid sequence—Metamyelocyte

METAMYELOCYTE

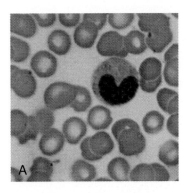

Figure 5–8A Metamyelocyte

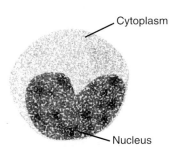

Figure 5–8B Schematic of metamyelocyte

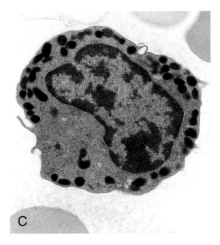

Figure 5–8C Electron micrograph of metamyelocyte (×22,250)

SIZE: 10–15μ
NUCLEUS: Indented
    Nucleoli: Not visible
    Chromatin: Coarse clumped
CYTOPLASM: Pale blue to pink
    Granules:
        Primary: Few
        Secondary: Many (full complement)

N/C RATIO: 1.5:1
REFERENCE INTERVAL:
    Bone Marrow: 13–22%
    Peripheral Blood: 0%

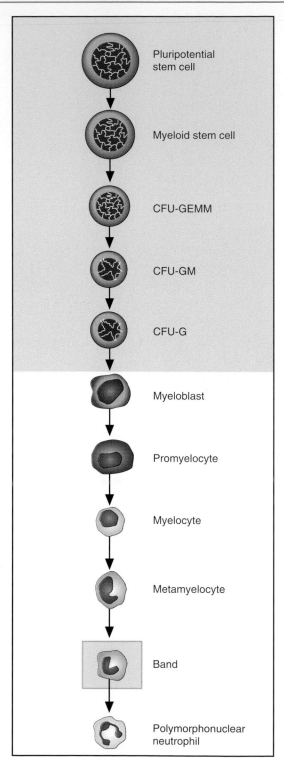

Figure 5–9 Myeloid sequence—Band

BAND

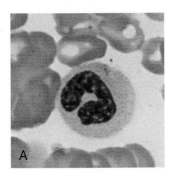

Figure 5–10A   Band

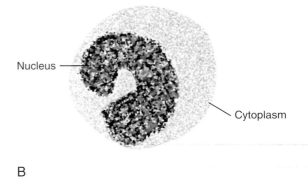

Figure 5–10B   Schematic of band

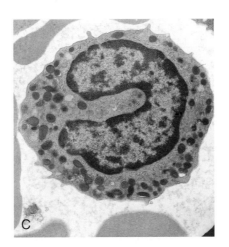

Figure 5–10C   Electron micrograph
of band (×22,250)

SIZE: 10–15μ

NUCLEUS: Band shaped. Constricted but no
threadlike filament. (NOTE:
Chromatin must be visible in
constriction.)
Nucleoli: Not visible
Chromatin: Coarse clumped

CYTOPLASM: Pale blue to pink
Granules:
Primary: Few
Secondary: Abundant
N/C RATIO: Cytoplasm predominates
REFERENCE INTERVAL:
Bone Marrow: 17–33%
Peripheral Blood: 0–5%

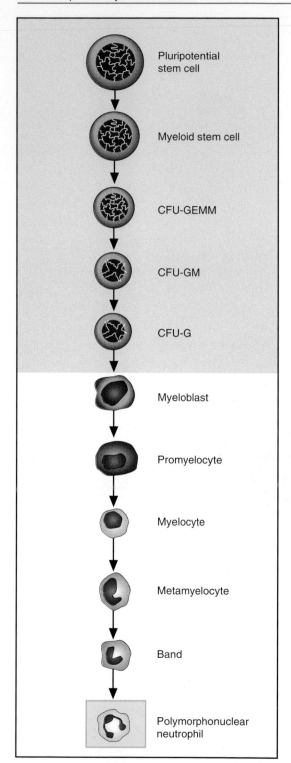

Pluripotential stem cell

Myeloid stem cell

CFU-GEMM

CFU-GM

CFU-G

Myeloblast

Promyelocyte

Myelocyte

Metamyelocyte

Band

Polymorphonuclear neutrophil

Figure 5–11 Myeloid sequence—Polymorphonuclear neutrophil

POLYMORPHONUCLEAR NEUTROPHIL (PMN)

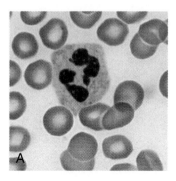

Figure 5–12A
Polymorphonuclear
neutrophil

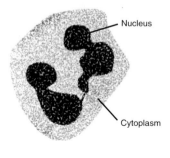

Figure 5–12B Schematic of
polymorphonuclear
neutrophil

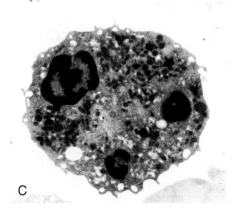

Figure 5–12C Electron micrograph of
polymorphonuclear neutrophil (×22,250)

SIZE: 10–15µ
NUCLEUS: 2–5 lobes connected by thin fila-
ments without visible chromatin
    Nucleoli: Not visible
    Chromatin: Coarse clumped
CYTOPLASM: Pale blue to pink
    Granules:
        Primary: Rare
        Secondary: Abundant

N/C RATIO: Cytoplasm predominates
REFERENCE INTERVAL:
    Bone Marrow: 3–11%
    Peripheral Blood: 50–70%

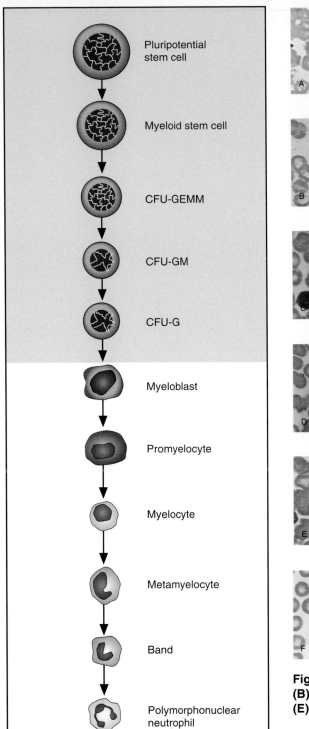

Pluripotential stem cell

Myeloid stem cell

CFU-GEMM

CFU-GM

CFU-G

Myeloblast

Promyelocyte

Myelocyte

Metamyelocyte

Band

Polymorphonuclear neutrophil

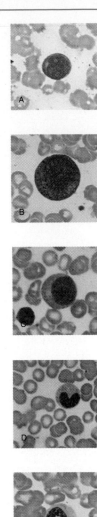

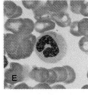

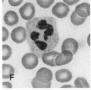

Figure 5–13   Myeloid sequence with **(A)** myeloblast, **(B)** promyelocyte, **(C)** myelocyte, **(D)** metamyelocyte, **(E)** band, and **(F)** polymorphonuclear neutrophil

6

Monocyte Maturation

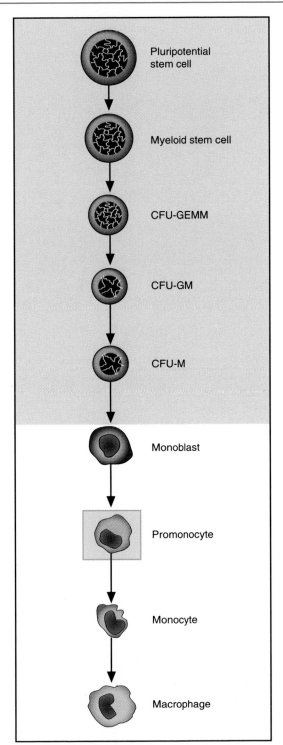

Pluripotential
stem cell

Myeloid stem cell

CFU-GEMM

CFU-GM

CFU-M

Monoblast

Promonocyte

Monocyte

Macrophage

Figure 6–1 Monocyte sequence—Promonocyte

NOTE: It is difficult to identify a monoblast morphologically with a high degree of certainty. Therefore, a photomicrograph of a monoblast is not included in this atlas.

PROMONOCYTE

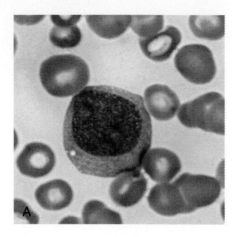

Figure 6–2A   Promonocyte

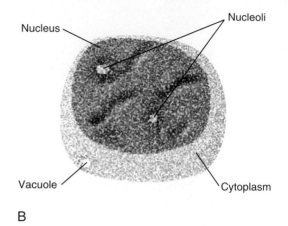

Figure 6–2B   Schematic of promonocyte

SIZE: 12–20μ
NUCLEUS: Irregularly shaped; deeply indented
    Nucleoli: May or may not be visible
    Chromatin: Fine
CYTOPLASM: Blue to gray
    Granules: Fine azurophilic
N/C RATIO: 2–3:1
REFERENCE INTERVAL:
    Bone Marrow: <1%
    Peripheral Blood: 0%

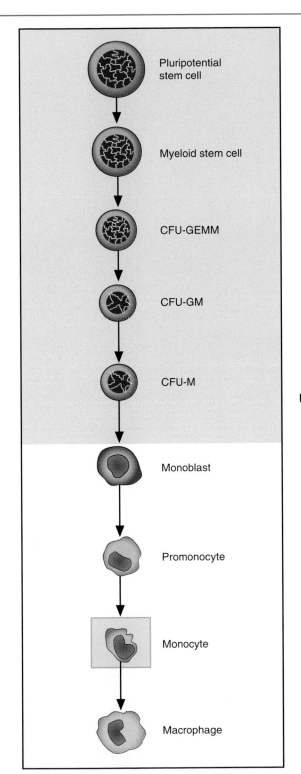

Figure 6–3 Monocyte sequence—Monocyte

MONOCYTE

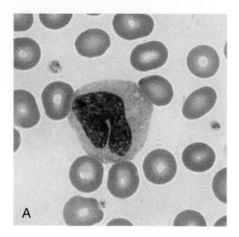

Figure 6–4A   Monocyte

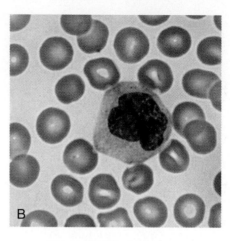

Figure 6–4B   Monocyte

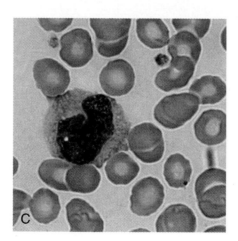

Figure 6–4C   Monocyte

SIZE: 12–20μ

NUCLEUS: Variable; may be round, horse-shoe- or kidney-shaped. Often has folds producing "brainlike" convolutions.

Nucleoli: Not visible

Chromatin: Lacy

CYTOPLASM: Blue-gray; may have pseudopods

Granules: Many fine granules frequently giving the appearance of ground glass

Vacuoles: Absent to numerous

N/C RATIO: Variable

REFERENCE INTERVAL:

Bone Marrow: 2%

Peripheral Blood: 3–11%

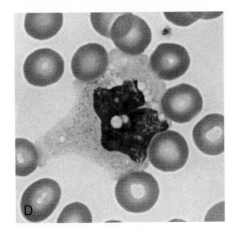

Figure 6–4D   Monocyte

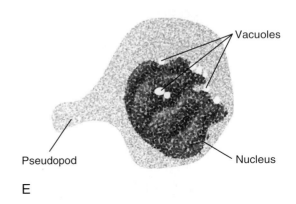

Figure 6–4E   Schematic of monocyte

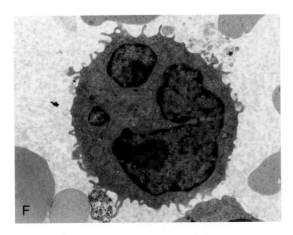

Figure 6–4F   Electron micrograph of monocyte (×16,500)

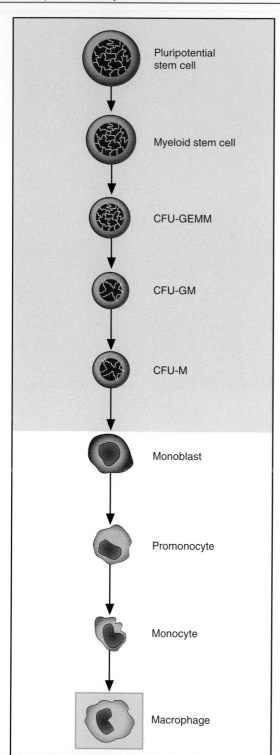

Figure 6–5   Monocyte sequence—Macrophage

MACROPHAGE

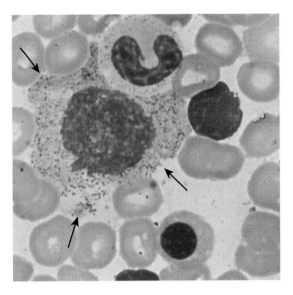

Figure 6–6 Macrophage

SIZE: 15–80 μm
NUCLEUS: Eccentric, reniform, egg-shaped, indented, or elongated
    Nucleoli: 1–2
    Chromatin: Fine, dispersed
CYTOPLASM: Abundant with irregular borders; may contain ingested material
    Granules: Many coarse azurophilic
    Vacuoles: May be present
REFERENCE INTERVAL: NA

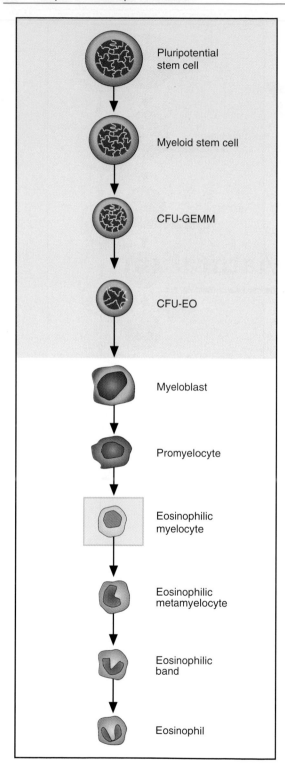

Figure 7–1 Eosinophilic sequence—Eosinophilic myelocyte

EOSINOPHILIC MYELOCYTE

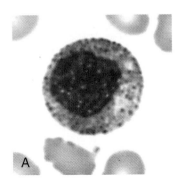

Figure 7–2A Eosinophilic myelocyte

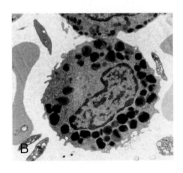

Figure 7–2B Electron micrograph of eosinophilic myelocyte

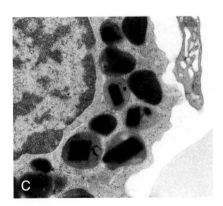

Figure 7–2C Electron micrograph of eosinophilic granule to demonstrate internal structures

SIZE: 12–18μ
NUCLEUS: Round to oval; may have one flattened side
    Nucleoli: Usually not visible
    Chromatin: Coarse and more condensed than promyelocyte
CYTOPLASM: Colorless to pink
    Granules:
        Primary: Few to moderate
        Secondary: Variable number; orange to red; round
N/C RATIO: 2:1
REFERENCE INTERVAL:
    Bone Marrow: 0–2%
    Peripheral Blood: 0%

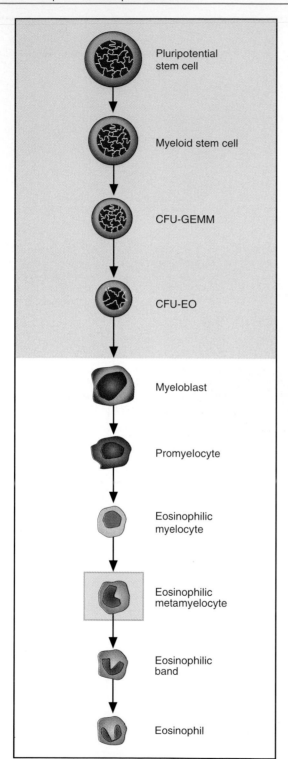

Pluripotential stem cell

Myeloid stem cell

CFU-GEMM

CFU-EO

Myeloblast

Promyelocyte

Eosinophilic myelocyte

Eosinophilic metamyelocyte

Eosinophilic band

Eosinophil

Figure 7–3 Eosinophilic sequence—Eosinophilic metamyelocyte

EOSINOPHILIC METAMYELOCYTE

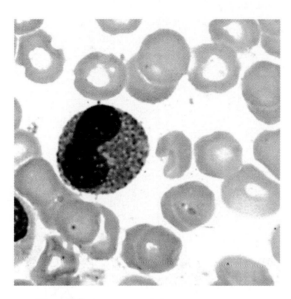

Figure 7–4   Eosinophilic metamyelocyte

SIZE: 10–15µ
NUCLEUS: Indented
    Nucleoli: Not visible
    Chromatin: Coarse clumped
CYTOPLASM: Colorless to pink
    Granules:
        Primary: Few
        Secondary: Many red to orange; round
N/C RATIO: 1.5:1
REFERENCE INTERVAL:
    Bone Marrow: 0–2%
    Peripheral Blood: 0%

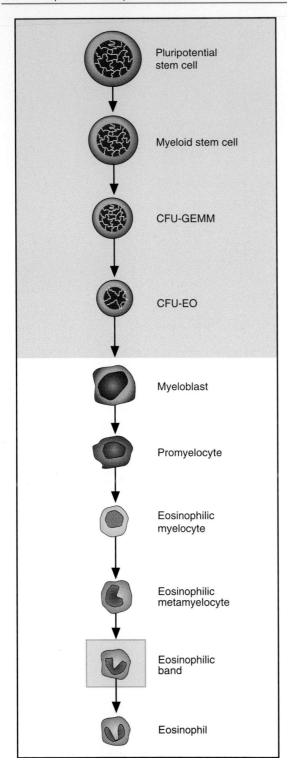

Pluripotential
stem cell

Myeloid stem cell

CFU-GEMM

CFU-EO

Myeloblast

Promyelocyte

Eosinophilic
myelocyte

Eosinophilic
metamyelocyte

Eosinophilic
band

Eosinophil

Figure 7–5   Eosinophilic sequence—Eosinophilic band

EOSINOPHILIC BAND

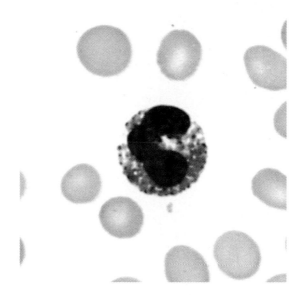

Figure 7–6   Eosinophilic band

SIZE: 10 15μ
NUCLEUS: Band shaped. Constricted but no threadlike filament. (NOTE: Chromatin must be
        visible in constriction.)
    Nucleoli: Not visible
    Chromatin: Coarse clumped
CYTOPLASM: Colorless to pink
    Granules:
        Primary: Few
        Secondary: Abundant red to orange; round
N/C RATIO: Cytoplasm predominates
REFERENCE INTERVAL:
    Bone Marrow: 0–2%
    Peripheral Blood: Rarely seen

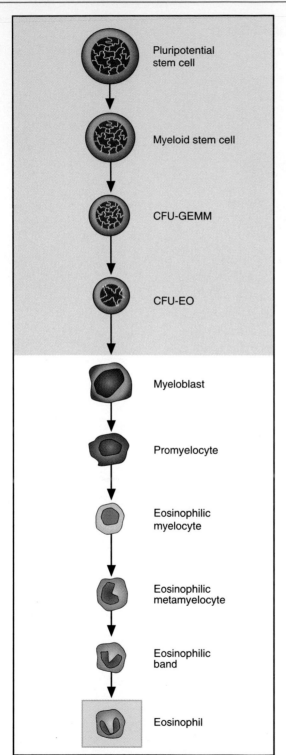

Figure 7–7   Eosinophilic sequence—Eosinophil

EOSINOPHIL

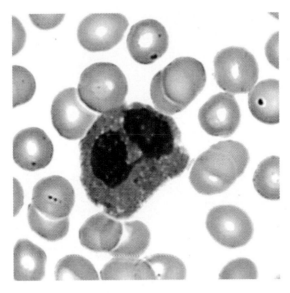

Figure 7–8 Eosinophil

SIZE: 12–17μ
NUCLEUS: 2–3 lobes connected by thin filaments without visible chromatin.
    Nucleoli: Not visible
    Chromatin: Coarse clumped
CYTOPLASM: Pink; may have irregular borders
    Granules:
        Primary: Rare
        Secondary: Abundant red to orange; round
N/C RATIO: Cytoplasm predominates
REFERENCE INTERVAL:
    Bone Marrow: 0–3%
    Peripheral Blood: 0–5%

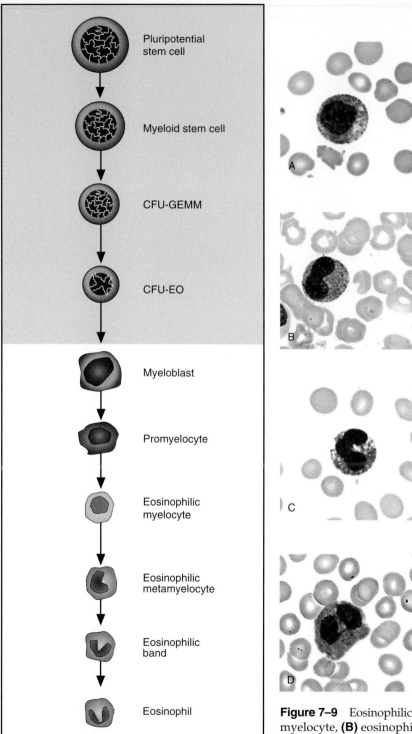

Figure 7–9 Eosinophilic sequence with **(A)** eosinophilic myelocyte, **(B)** eosinophilic metamyelocyte, **(C)** eosinophilic band, and **(D)** eosinophil

CHAPTER 8

Basophil Maturation

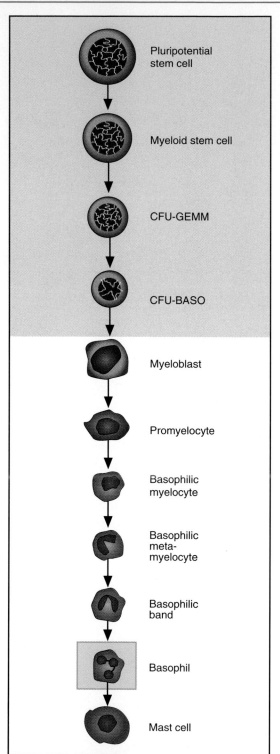

Figure 8–1 Basophilic sequence—Basophil

BASOPHIL

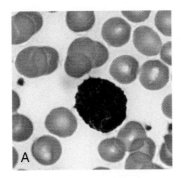

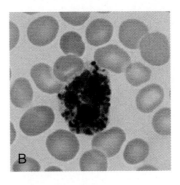

Figure 8–2A   Basophil   **Figure 8–2B**   Basophil

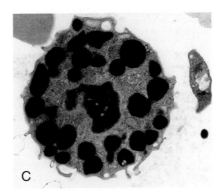

Figure 8–2C   Electron micrograph
of basophil (×28,750)

SIZE: 10–14μ
NUCLEUS: Usually 2 lobes connected by thin filaments without visible chromatin
    Nucleoli: Not visible
    Chromatin: Coarse clumped
CYTOPLASM: Lavender to colorless
    Granules:
        Primary: Rare
        Secondary: Variable in number with uneven distribution, may obscure nucleus **(A);**
                deep purple to black; irregularly shaped. Granules are water soluble and
                may be washed out during staining; thus, they appear as empty areas in
                the cytoplasm **(B).**
N/C RATIO: Cytoplasm predominates.
REFERENCE INTERVAL:
    Bone Marrow: <1%
    Peripheral Blood: 0–1%

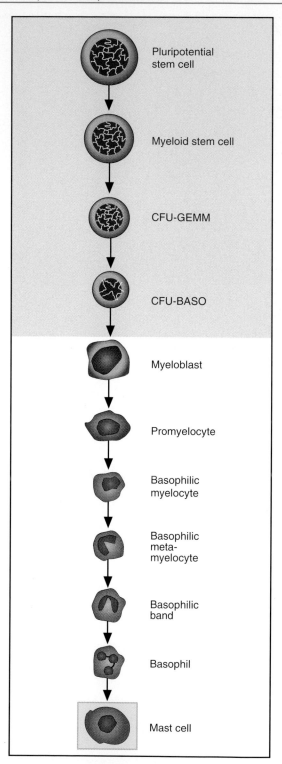

Pluripotential stem cell

Myeloid stem cell

CFU-GEMM

CFU-BASO

Myeloblast

Promyelocyte

Basophilic myelocyte

Basophilic meta-myelocyte

Basophilic band

Basophil

Mast cell

Figure 8–3   Basophilic sequence—Mast cell

MAST CELL

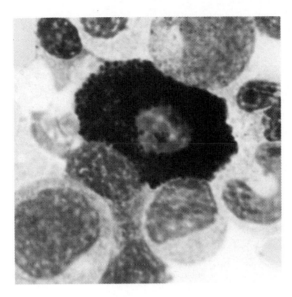

Figure 8–4   Mast cell

SIZE: 12–25μ
NUCLEUS: Round to oval, centrally located, may be obscured by granules
CYTOPLASM: Lavender to colorless
    Granules: Many dark blue to black
REFERENCE INTERVAL:
    Bone Marrow: <1%
    Peripheral Blood: None

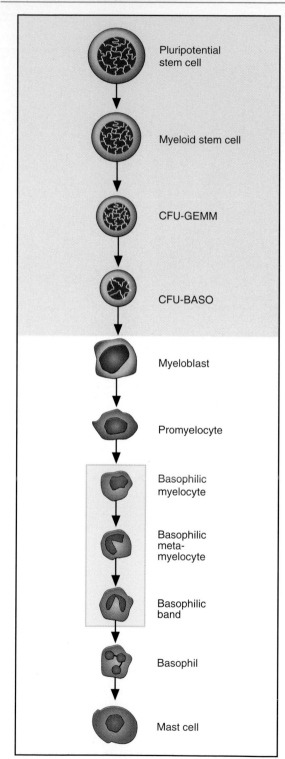

Pluripotential stem cell

Myeloid stem cell

CFU-GEMM

CFU-BASO

Myeloblast

Promyelocyte

Basophilic myelocyte

Basophilic meta-myelocyte

Basophilic band

Basophil

Mast cell

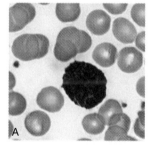

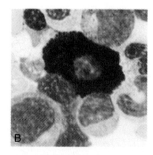

Figure 8–5 Maturation parallels that of the neutrophil; however, immature stages are extremely rare. **(A)** Basophil, **(B)** mast cell.

9

Lymphoid Maturation

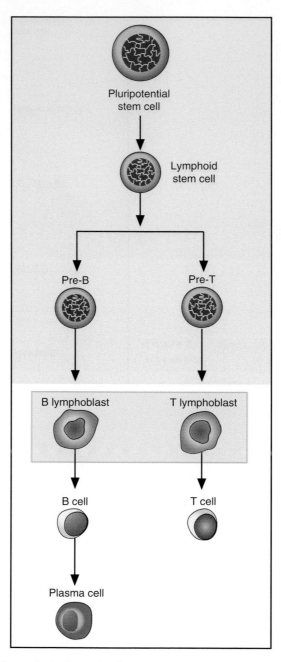

Figure 9–1 Lymphoid sequence—B lymphoblast and T lymphoblast

LYMPHOBLAST

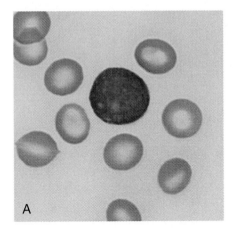

Figure 9–2A   Lymphoblast

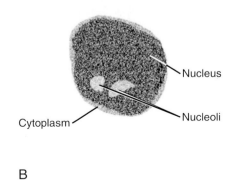

B

Figure 9–2B   Schematic of lymphoblast

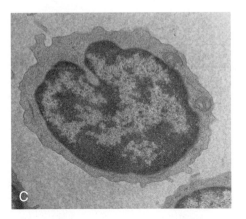

Figure 9–2C   Electron micrograph of lymphoblast (×28,750)

SIZE: 10–18μ
NUCLEUS: Round to oval
    Nucleoli: One or more
    Chromatin: Fine, evenly stained
CYTOPLASM: Moderate to deeply basophilic
    Granules: None
N/C RATIO: 4:1
REFERENCE INTERVAL:
    Bone Marrow: Not defined
    Peripheral Blood: 0%

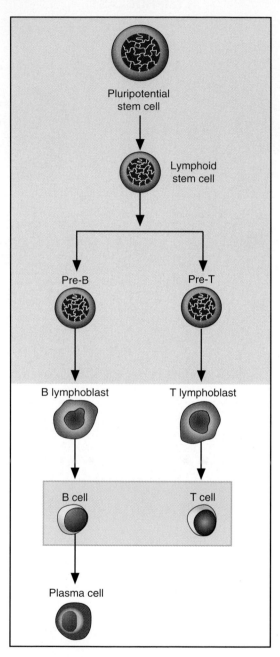

Figure 9–3 Lymphoid sequence—B and T cells
(NOTE: T lymphocytes cannot be distinguished from
B lymphocytes with Wright's stain)

LYMPHOCYTE

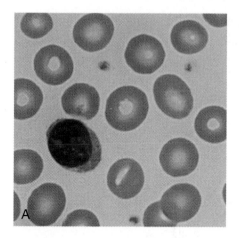

Figure 9–4A Small lymphocyte

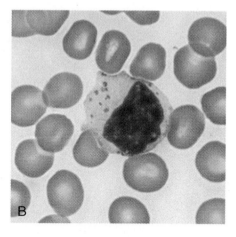

Figure 9–4B Large lymphocyte

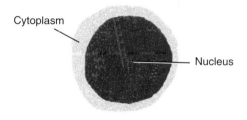

C

Figure 9–4C Schematic of lymphocyte

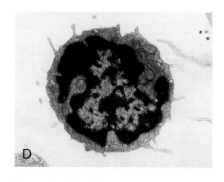

Figure 9–4D Electron micrograph of lymphocyte (×30,000)

SIZE: 7–18μ

NUCLEUS: Round to oval; may be slightly indented

    Nucleoli: Occasional

    Chromatin: Condensed to deeply condensed

CYTOPLASM: Scant to moderate; sky blue; vacuoles may be present (NOTE: The difference in size from small to large lymphocytes is due primarily to a larger amount of cytoplasm.)

    Granules: Few azurophilic

N/C RATIO: 3–5:1

REFERENCE INTERVAL:

    Bone Marrow: 5–15%

    Peripheral Blood: 20–40%

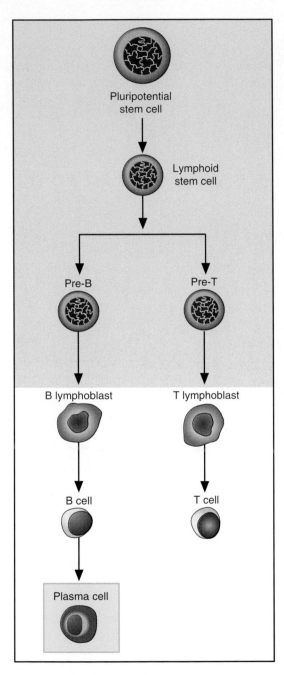

Figure 9–5   Lymphoid sequence—plasma cell

PLASMA CELL

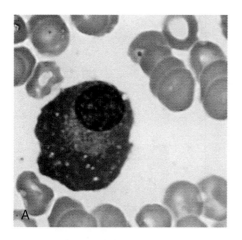

Figure 9–6A Plasma cell

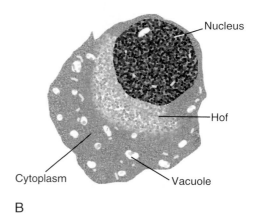

Figure 9–6B Schematic of plasma cell

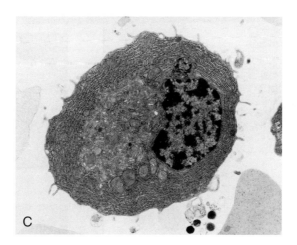

Figure 9–6C Electron micrograph of plasma cell (×17,500)

SIZE: 8–20μ
NUCLEUS: Round or oval; eccentric
    Nucleoli: None
    Chromatin: Coarse
CYTOPLASM: Deeply basophilic, often with
    perinuclear clear zone (hof)
    Granules: None
    Vacuoles: None to several

N/C RATIO: 2–1:1
REFERENCE INTERVAL:
    Bone Marrow: 0–1%
    Peripheral Blood: 0%

VARIATIONS IN SIZE

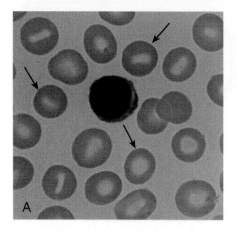

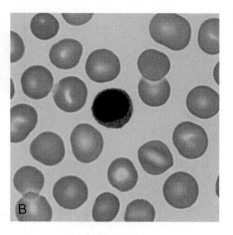

Figure 10–1A   Microcytes

Associated with: Iron deficiency anemia
Sideroblastic anemia
Thalassemia minor
Chronic disease
(occasionally)
Lead poisoning
Hemoglobinopathies
(some)

Figure 10–1B   Normocytes

Normal erythrocytes are
approximately the same size as the
nucleus of a small lymphocyte.

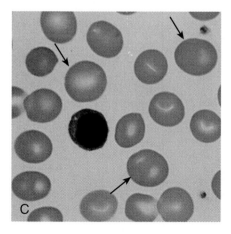

Figure 10–1C   Macrocytes

Associated with: Liver disease
Vitamin B_{12} deficiency
Folate deficiency
Neonates

DIMORPHIC POPULATION OF ERYTHROCYTES

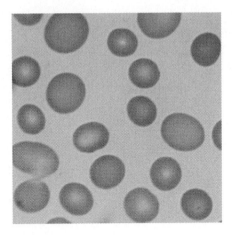

Figure 10–2   Dimorphic population of erythrocytes

Associated with: Transfusion
Myelodysplastic syndromes
Vitamin B_{12}, folate, or iron
deficiencies—early in treatment process

HEMOGLOBIN CONTENT OF ERYTHROCYTES

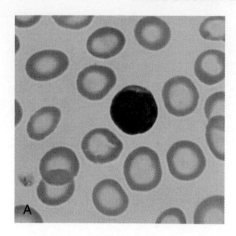

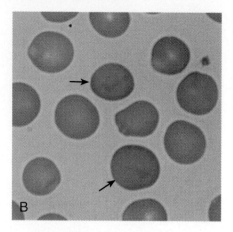

Figure 10–3A   Hypochromia

Associated with: Iron deficiency
                   anemia
                   Thalassemias
                   Sideroblastic anemia
                   Lead poisoning
                   Some cases of chronic
                   disease

NOTE: The central pallor zone of the
erythrocyte must be greater than one
third of the diameter of the cell
before it is classified as hypochromic. The cells in this figure are
also microcytic.

Figure 10–3B   Polychromasia

Associated with: Acute and chronic hemorrhage
                   Hemolysis
                   Effective treatment for anemia
                   Neonates

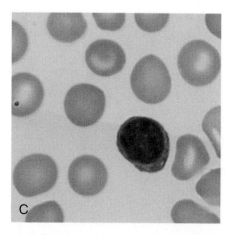

Figure 10–3C   Normochromic erythrocytes
For comparison with hypochromic and polychromatic erythrocytes

11

Variations in Shape and Color of Erythrocytes

ACANTHOCYTE
Spur Cell

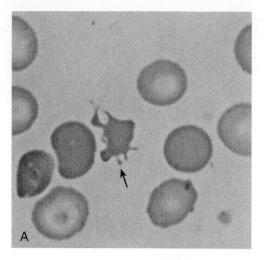

Figure 11–1A   Acanthocyte

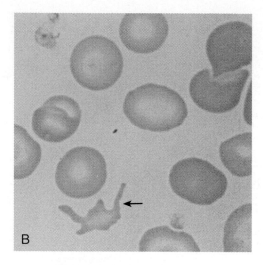

Figure 11–1B   Acanthocyte

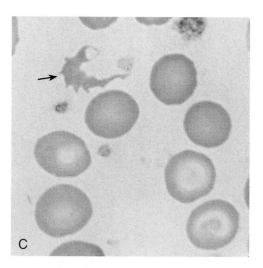

Figure 11–1C   Acanthocyte

Description: Erythrocyte with irregularly spaced projections that vary in width, length, and number

Associated with: Abetalipoproteinemia, severe liver disease, splenectomy, malabsorption, hypothyroidism, vitamin E deficiency

ECHINOCYTE
Burr Cell or Crenated Cell

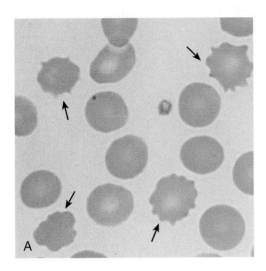

Figure 11–2A   Echinocytes

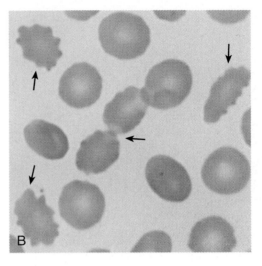

Figure 11–2B   Echinocytes

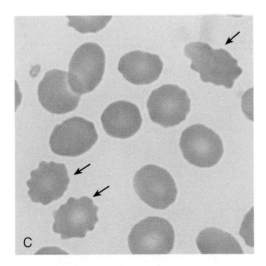

Figure 11–2C   Echinocytes

Description: Burrlike erythrocyte with short, evenly spaced projections

Associated with: Uremia, pryuvate kinase deficiency, microangiopathic hemolytic anemia, artifact

SPHEROCYTE

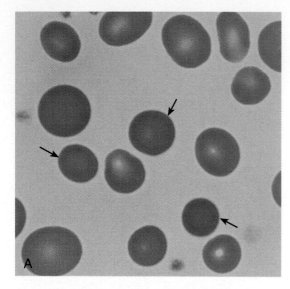

Figure 11–3A   Spherocytes   **Figure 11–3B**   Spherocytes

COLOR: Dark red
SHAPE: Round; no central pallor zone
Associated with: Hereditary spherocytosis, some hemolytic anemias, transfused cells, severe
                   burns

CODOCYTE
Target Cell

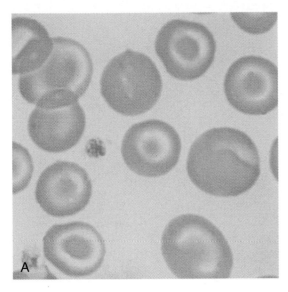

Figure 11–4A   Codocytes

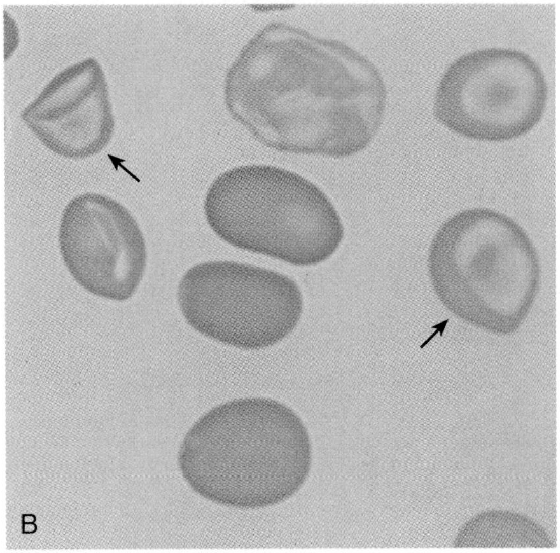

Figure 11–4B   Codocytes

COLOR: Red to salmon

SHAPE: Bull's eye; central concentration of hemoglobin surrounded by colorless area with peripheral ring of hemoglobin resembling bull's eye; may be bell shaped.

Associated with: Hemoglobinopathies, thalassemia, iron deficiency anemia, splenectomy, obstructive liver disease

DREPANOCYTE
Sickle Cell

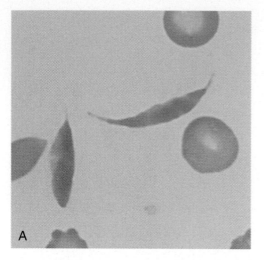

Figure 11–5A   Drepanocyte

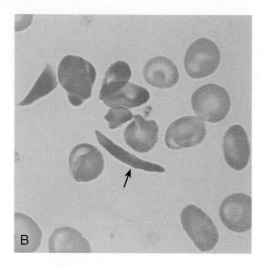

Figure 11–5B   Drepanocyte

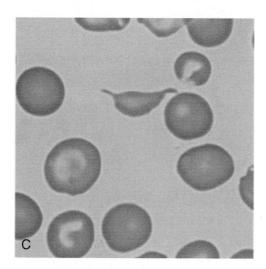

Figure 11–5C   Schizocyte resembling drepanocyte

COLOR: Dark red to salmon
SHAPE: Elongated cell with point on each end; may be curved or S-shaped
COMPOSITION: Hemoglobin S
Associated with: Homozygous hemoglobin S disease

HEMOGLOBIN C CRYSTALS

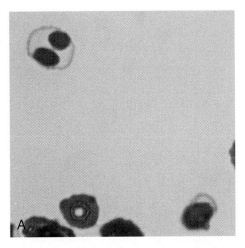

Figure 11–6A   Induced hemoglobin C crystals (crystals induced with 3% NaCl)

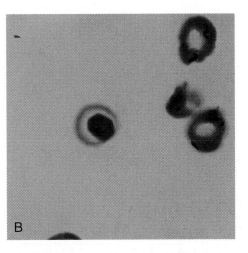

Figure 11–6B   Induced hemoglobin C crystal (crystals induced with 3% NaCl)

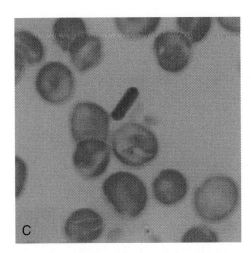

Figure 11–6C   Hemoglobin C crystal (not induced on peripheral blood smear)

COLOR: Dark red
SHAPE: Hexagonal
NUMBER PER CELL: 1 (if not induced)
COMPOSITION: Hemoglobin C
Associated with: Homozygous hemoglobin C disease

HEMOGLOBIN SC CRYSTALS

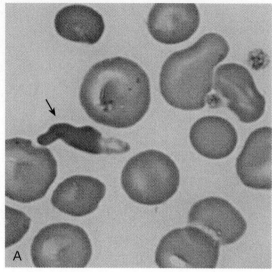

Figure 11–7A   Hemoglobin SC crystal

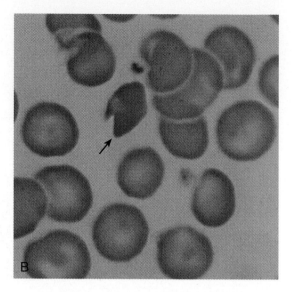

Figure 11–7B   Hemoglobin SC crystal

COLOR: Dark red
SHAPE: 1–2 finger-like projections; may look like a mitten
NUMBER PER CELL: 1–2
COMPOSITION: Hemoglobin SC
Associated with: Hemoglobin SC disease

STOMATOCYTE

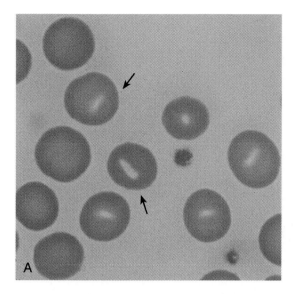

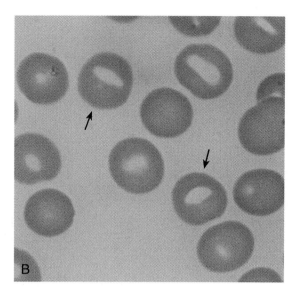

Figure 11–8A   Stomatocytes   **Figure 11–8B**   Stomatocytes

Description: Erythrocyte with slit-like area of central pallor
Associated with: Hereditary stomatocytosis, alcoholism, liver disease, Rh null phenotype, artifact

SCHIZOCYTE
Schistocyte

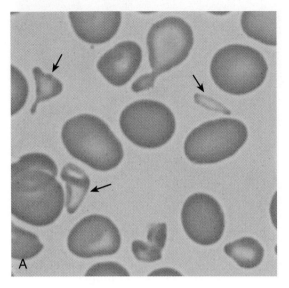

Figure 11–11A   Schizocytes   **Figure 11–11B**   Schizocytes

COLOR: Red to salmon
SHAPE: Fragmented erythrocytes; many sizes and shapes are present on a smear; often display
          pointed extremities
Associated with: Microangiopathic hemolytic anemia (disseminated intravascular coagulation),
          severe burns, hemolytic-uremic syndrome, thrombotic thrombocytopenic
          purpura, renal graft rejection

ROULEAUX VS AUTOAGGLUTINATION

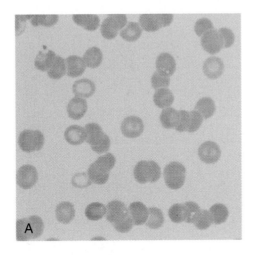

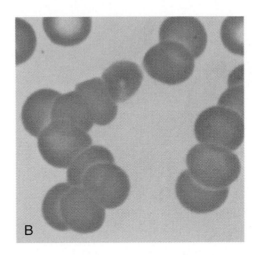

Figure 11–12A   Rouleaux (×500)   **Figure 11–12B**   Rouleaux (×1000)

Description: Erythrocytes arranged in rows like stacks of coins
Associated with: Increased concentrations of globulins and/or paraproteins

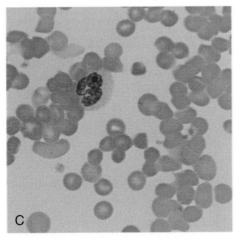

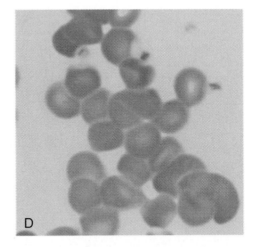

Figure 11–12C   Autoagglutination (×500)   **Figure 11–12D**   Autoagglutination (×1000)

Description: Clumping of erythrocytes; outlines of individual cells may not be evident
Associated with: Antigen/antibody reactions

CHAPTER

12

Inclusions in Erythrocytes

Table 12–1   STAINING QUALITIES OF ERYTHROCYTE INCLUSION BODIES

Inclusion	Wright-Giemsa stain	New Methylene Blue (or Other Supravital Stain)	Prussian Blue (Iron)
Howell-Jolly body	+	+	0
Basophilic stippling	+	+	0
Pappenheimer body	+	+	+
Cabot ring	+	+	0
Reticulocyte	0	+	0
Heinz body	0	+	0

HOWELL-JOLLY BODIES

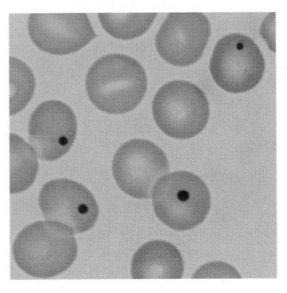

Figure 12–1 Howell-Jolly bodies

COLOR: Dark blue to purple
SHAPE: Round to oval
SIZE: 1μ
NUMBER PER CELL: Usually 1; may be multiple
COMPOSITION: DNA
Associated with: Splenectomy, hyposplenism, megaloblastic anemia, hemolytic anemia

BASOPHILIC STIPPLING

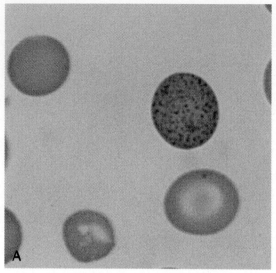

Figure 12–2A Basophilic stippling

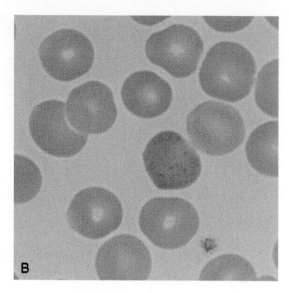

Figure 12–2B Basophilic stippling

COLOR: Dark blue to purple
SHAPE: Fine or coarse granules
NUMBER PER CELL: Numerous with fairly even distribution
COMPOSITION: RNA
Associated with: Lead intoxication, thalassemia, abnormal heme synthesis

PAPPENHEIMER BODIES
Siderotic Granules

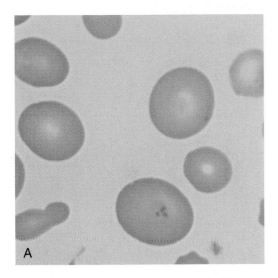

Figure 12–3A   Pappenheimer bodies

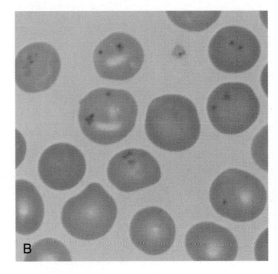

Figure 12–3B   Pappenheimer bodies

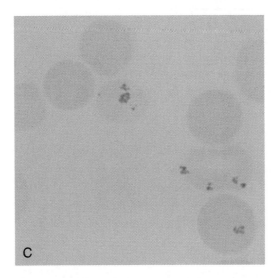

Figure 12–3C   Siderotic granules—iron stain

COLOR: Light blue

SHAPE: Fine irregular granules in clusters

NUMBER PER CELL: Usually one cluster; may be multiples. Often at periphery of cell.

COMPOSITION: Iron

Associated with: Splenectomy, hemolytic anemia, sideroblastic anemia, megaloblastic anemia, hemoglobinopathies

CABOT RING

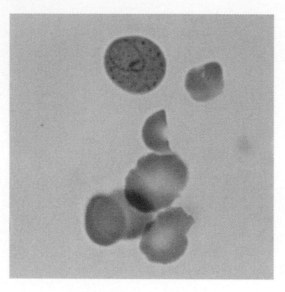

Figure 12–4   Cabot ring

COLOR: Dark blue to purple
SHAPE: Loop, ring, or figure eight; may look like beads on a string
NUMBER PER CELL: 1–2
COMPOSITION: Thought to be remnants of mitotic spindle
Associated with: Myelodysplastic syndrome, megaloblastic anemia

COMPARISON OF RETICULOCYTES AND HEINZ BODIES
Stained with New Methylene Blue

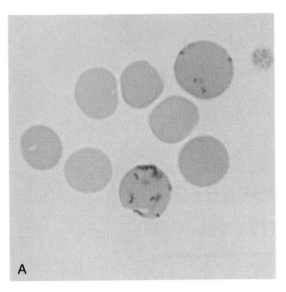

Figure 12–5A   Reticulocytes

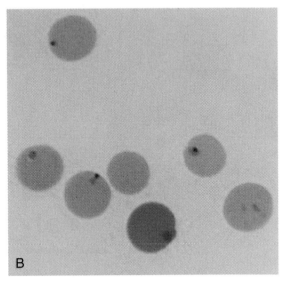

Figure 12–5B   Heinz bodies

CELL: Anuclear immature erythrocyte
COMPOSITION: Precipitated RNA
NUMBER: ≥2/cell
COLOR: Dark blue
Associated with: Erythrocyte maturation

CELL: Mature erythrocyte
COMPOSITION: Precipitated hemoglobin
NUMBER: Single or multiple, generally membrane bound
COLOR: Dark blue to purple
Associated with: Unstable hemoglobin, some hemoglobinopathies, some erythrocyte enzyme deficiencies
NOTE: To stimulate the formation of Heinz bodies in susceptible cells, blood may be incubated with acetylphenylhydrazine.

IRON DEFICIENCY ANEMIA

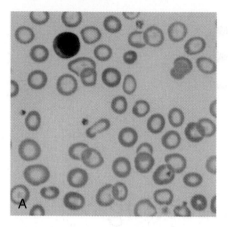

Figure 13–1A   Iron deficiency anemia (peripheral blood [PB] ×500)

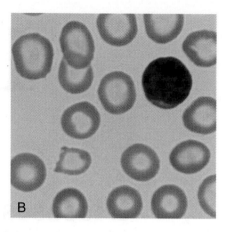

Figure 13–1B   Iron deficiency anemia (PB ×1000)

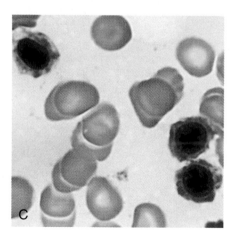

Figure 13–1C   Iron deficiency anemia (bone marrow [BM] ×1000) (showing shaggy cytoplasm)

Peripheral blood: Erythrocytes are hypochromic and microcytic; large variation in size; possible thrombocytosis

Bone marrow: Erythrocyte precursors are smaller and more numerous than normal and have shaggy cytoplasm. There is nuclear cytoplasmic asynchrony, with cytoplasmic maturation lagging behind that of the nucleus. Although characteristic findings for disease states are listed, not all may be present in one patient. The most common ones are depicted.

α AND β THALASSEMIA MINOR

$$--/\alpha\alpha \qquad -\alpha/-\alpha \qquad -/\alpha\alpha$$
$$\beta/\beta^0 \quad \beta/\beta^+ \quad \beta/(\delta\beta)^0 \qquad \beta/(\delta\beta)\textbf{Lepore}$$

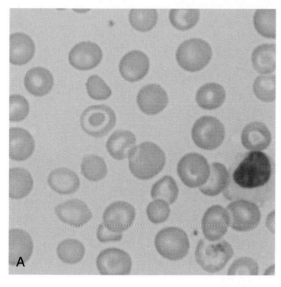

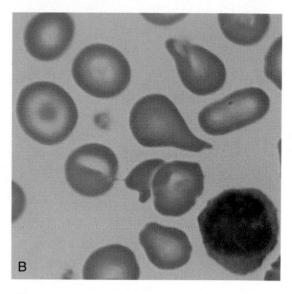

Figure 13–2A Thalassemia minor (PB ×500)   **Figure 13–2B** Thalassemia minor (PB ×1000)

Peripheral blood: Microcytosis, slight hypochromia, codocytes, basophilic stippling

β-THALASSEMIA MAJOR

$β^0β^0$ $β^+β^+$ $β^0β^+$ **(δβ)Lepore/(δβ)Lepore**

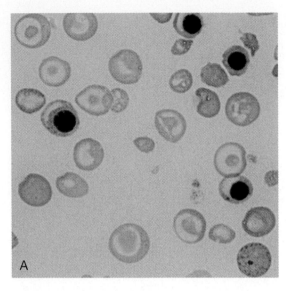

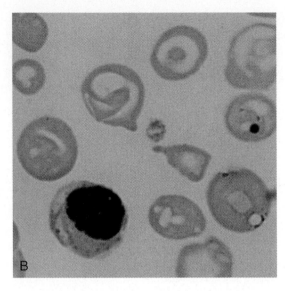

Figure 13–3A   β-Thalassemia major (PB ×500)

Figure 13–3B   β-Thalassemia major (PB ×1000)

Peripheral Blood: Numerous nucleated erythrocytes, microcytes, hypochromia, codocytes, basophilic stippling, many dacryocytes, many schizocytes, polychromasia

BART'S HEMOGLOBIN
(4 α − Chain Deletion)

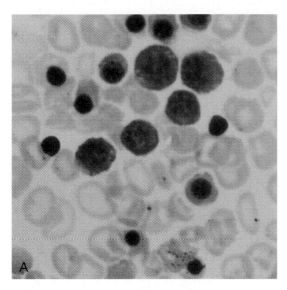

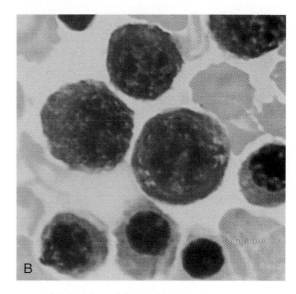

Figure 13–4A Bart's hemoglobin (PB ×500)   **Figure 13–4B** Bart's hemoglobin (PB ×1000)

Peripheral Blood: Marked variation in size, hypochromia, numerous nucleated erythrocytes, variable polychromasia, macrocytes

MACROCYTIC ANEMIA
Nonmegaloblastic

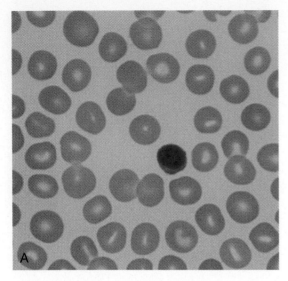

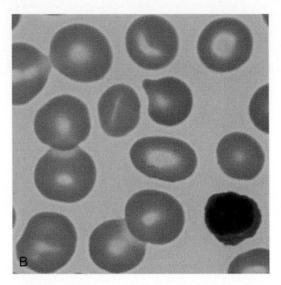

Figure 13–5A Macrocytic (nonmegaloblastic) (×500)

Figure 13–5B Macrocytic (nonmegaloblastic) (×1000)

Peripheral Blood: Round macrocytes (MCV = 112 fL), leukocyte and platelet counts usually normal

Bone marrow: No megaloblastic changes

MEGALOBLASTIC ANEMIA

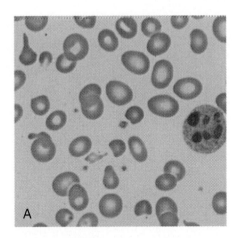

Figure 13–6A   Megaloblastic (PB ×500)

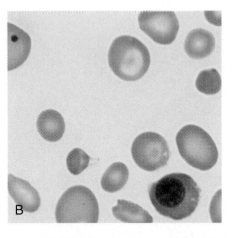

Figure 13–6B   Megaloblastic (PB ×1000)

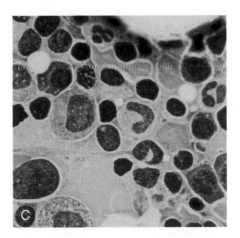

Figure 13–6C   Megaloblastic (BM ×500)

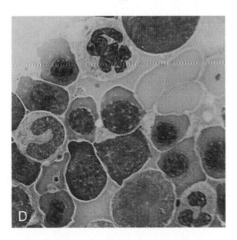

Figure 13–6D   Megaloblastic (BM ×1000)

Peripheral Blood: Pancytopenia, oval macrocytes, Howell-Jolly bodies, nucleated erythrocytes, basophilic stippling, hypersegmentation of neutrophils, giant platelets, codocytes, schizocytes, spherocytes, dacryocytes

NOTE: Triad of abnormalities: Oval macrocytes, hypersegmented neutrophils, and Howell-Jolly bodies

Bone Marrow: Hypercellular, asynchrony (trilineage), giant bands, giant metamyelocytes, hypersegmented megakaryocytes

APLASTIC ANEMIA

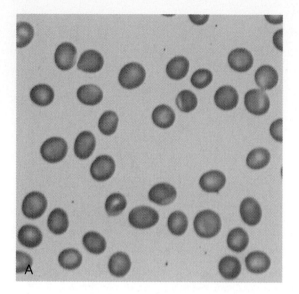

Figure 13–7A   Aplastic anemia (PB ×500)

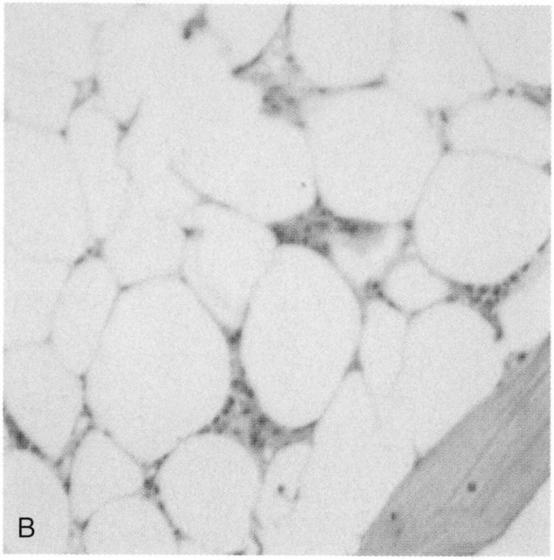

Figure 13–7B   Aplastic anemia (BM biopsy ×500)

Peripheral Blood: Pancytopenia, normocytic, normochromic (occasional macrocytes)
Bone Marrow: Hypocellular; lymphocytes may predominate

IMMUNE HEMOLYTIC ANEMIA

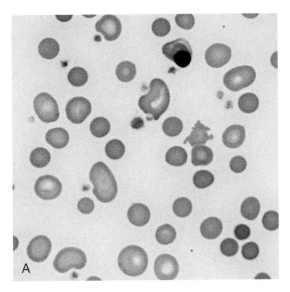

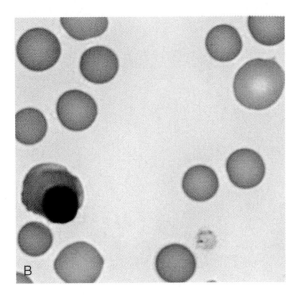

Figure 13–8A   Immune hemolytic anemia (PB ×500)

Figure 13–8B   Immune hemolytic anemia (PB ×1000)

Peripheral Blood: Spherocytes, schizocytes, polychromasia, nucleated erythrocytes

NOTE: Erythrocyte morphology varies with cause and severity of disease.

HEMOLYTIC DISEASE OF THE NEWBORN

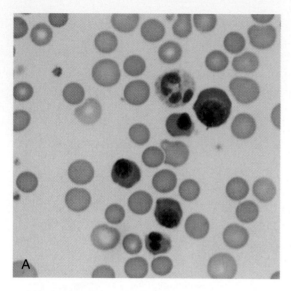

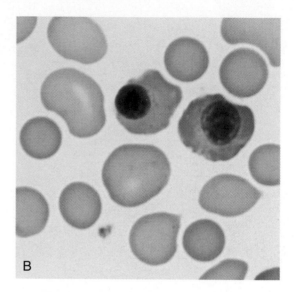

Figure 13–9A Hemolytic disease of the newborn (PB ×500)

Figure 13–9B Hemolytic disease of the newborn (PB ×1000)

Peripheral Blood: Increased number of nucleated erythrocytes, macrocytic/normochromic, polychromasia, spherocytes

NOTE: Normal newborns have some nucleated erythrocytes

HEREDITARY SPHEROCYTOSIS

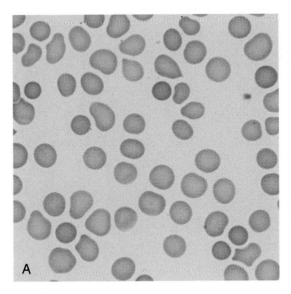

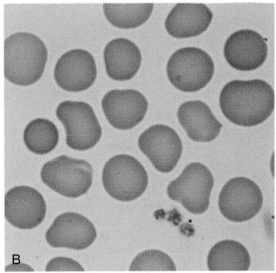

Figure 13–10A   Hereditary spherocytosis (PB ×500)

Figure 13–10B   Hereditary spherocytosis (PB ×1000)

Peripheral Blood: Spherocytes (variable in number), polychromasia; nucleated erythrocytes possible

HEREDITARY ELLIPTOCYTOSIS

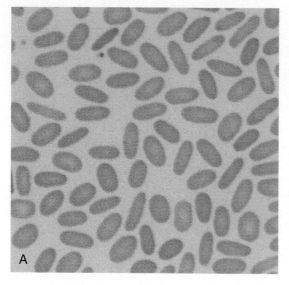

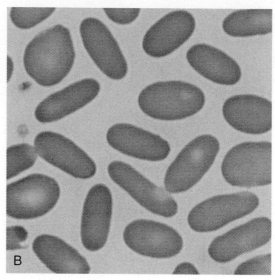

Figure 13–11A Hereditary elliptocytosis (PB ×500)

Figure 13–11B Hereditary elliptocytosis (PB ×1000)

Peripheral Blood: >25% elliptocytes, usually >60% elliptocytes; indices are normocytic, normochromic

NOTE: Hemolytic Variant of Hereditary Elliptocytosis: Microelliptocytes, schizocytes, spherocytes

MICROANGIOPATHIC HEMOLYTIC ANEMIA (MAHA)

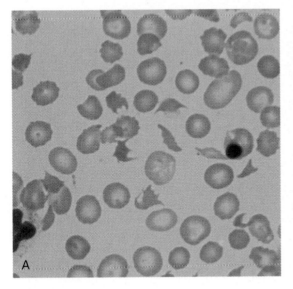 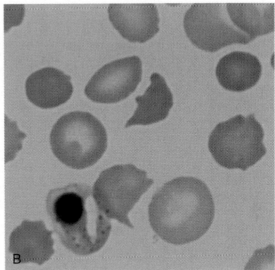

Figure 13–12A Microangiopathic hemolytic anemia (PB ×500)

Figure 13–12B Microangiopathic hemolytic anemia (PB ×1000)

Peripheral Blood: Schizocytes, spherocytes, polychromasia, nucleated erythrocytes, decreased platelet count

NOTE: The degree of morphologic change correlates directly with severity of the disease.

HEMOGLOBIN CC DISEASE

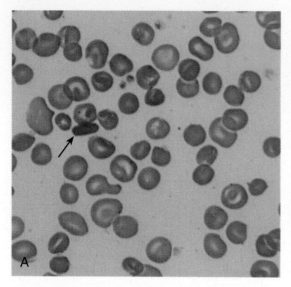 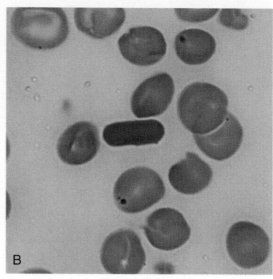

Figure 13–13A Hemoglobin CC (PB ×500)   **Figure 13–13B** Hemoglobin CC (PB ×1000)

Peripheral Blood: Codocytes, spherocytes, microcytes, polychromasia, intracellular or rod-shaped crystals possible

HEMOGLOBIN SS DISEASE

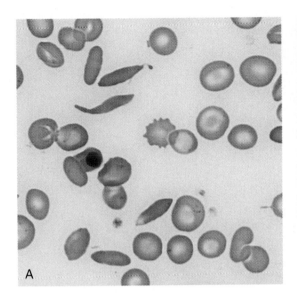

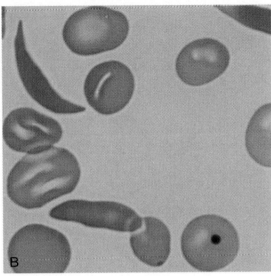

Figure 13–14A   Hemoglobin SS (PB ×500)   **Figure 13–14B**   Hemoglobin SS (PB ×1000)

Peripheral Blood: Drepanocytes (in crises), codocytes, nucleated erythrocytes, schizocytes, Howell-Jolly bodies, basophilic stippling, polychromasia, increased leukocyte count with neutrophilia, increased platelet count

14

Nuclear Alterations
of Leukocytes

HYPOSEGMENTATION

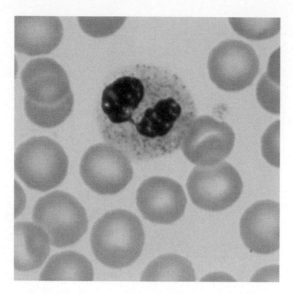

Figure 14–1   Hyposegmentation (PB ×1000)

Description: Bilobed or peanut-shaped neutrophil nucleus with coarse chromatin
Associated with: Pelger-Huët anomaly, myeloproliferative or myelodysplastic disorders

HYPERSEGMENTATION

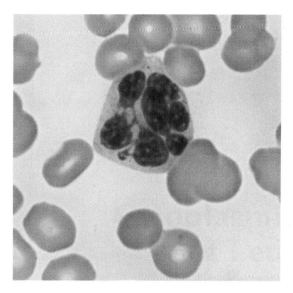

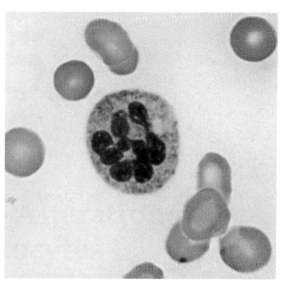

Figure 14–2A   Hypersegmentation (PB ×1000)   **Figure 14–2B**   Hypersegmentation (PB ×1000)

Description: Six or more lobes in neutrophil nucleus
Associated with: Megaloblastic anemias; chronic infections; rarely inherited

ERYTHROPHAGOCYTOSIS

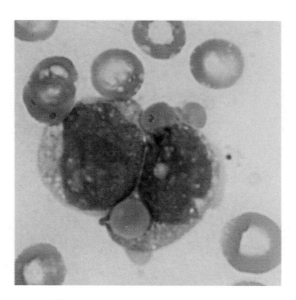

Figure 15–5 Erythrophagocytosis

Description: Monocyte or macrophage that has engulfed an erythrocyte

Associated with: Familial hemophagocytic histiocytosis; idiopathic

GAUCHER DISEASE

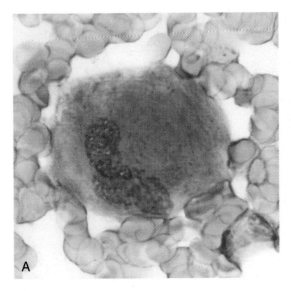

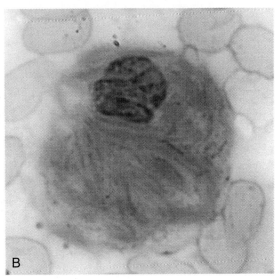

Figure 15–6A Gaucher disease   **Figure 15–6B** Gaucher disease

Description: The Gaucher cell is a macrophage 20–80μ in diameter with one or more small, round to oval eccentric nuclei; cytoplasm has crumpled tissue paper appearance. Found in bone marrow, spleen, liver, and other affected tissue.

NIEMANN-PICK DISEASE

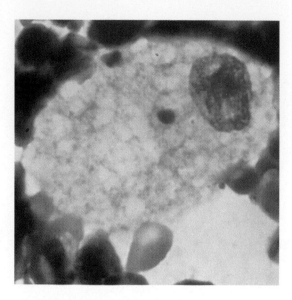

Figure 15–7 Niemann-Pick disease

Description: The Niemann-Pick cell is a macrophage, 20–90μ in diameter, with a small eccentric nucleus and foamy cytoplasm. It is found in bone marrow and lymphoid tissue. The peripheral blood of patients with Niemann-Pick disease may exhibit vacuolated lymphocytes.

SEA BLUE HISTIOCYTE

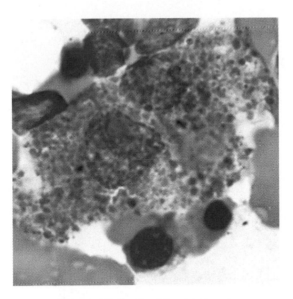

Figure 15–8 Sea blue histiocyte

Description: The sea blue histiocyte is a macrophage 20–60μ in diameter with an eccentric
nucleus. The cytoplasm contains varying numbers of prominent blue-green granules. These cells are found in spleen, liver, and bone marrow.

Associated with: Familial sea blue histiocytosis, myeloproliferative diseases

MAY-HEGGLIN ANOMALY

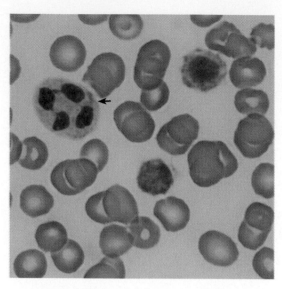

Figure 15–9   May-Hegglin anomaly

Description: This anomaly is characterized by thrombocytopenia with large and/or bizarre platelets and large inclusions resembling Döhle bodies in all leukocytes, with the absence of toxic granulation.

NOTE: These inclusions are sporadically visible by light microscopy but always detectable by electron microscopy.

CHÉDIAK-HIGASHI ANOMALY

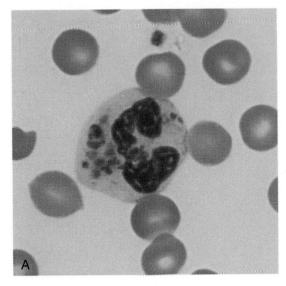

Figure 15–10A   Chédiak-Higashi anomaly; neutrophil with granules

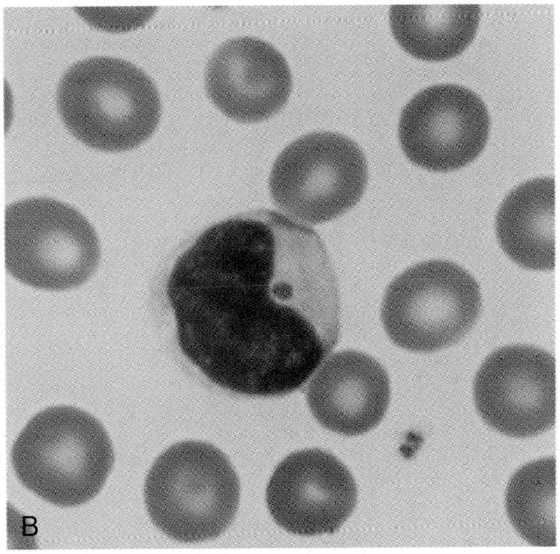

Figure 15–10B   Chédiak-Higashi anomaly; lymphocyte with granule

Description: Large gray-blue granules in the cytoplasm of many monocytes and granulocytes. Lymphocytes may contain large red-purple granules.

AUER RODS

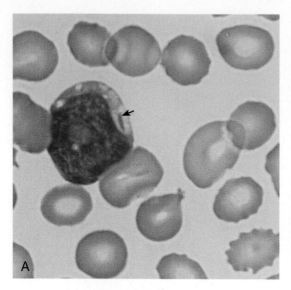

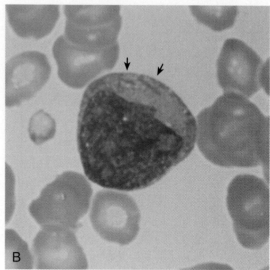

Figure 15–11A   Auer rod   **Figure 15–11B**   Auer rods

Description: Fused primary granules; usually rods; occasionally round

Color: Red

Location: Cytoplasm

Number: Single or multiple

Associated with: Acute leukemia—FAB* M1 through M6

*French-American-British classification of acute leukemia

REACTIVE LYMPHOCYTES

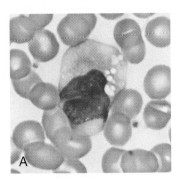

Figure 15–12A   Reactive lymphocyte, vacuolated cytoplasm

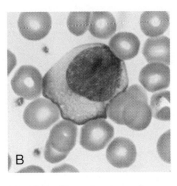

Figure 15–12B   Reactive lymphocyte, peripheral basophilia

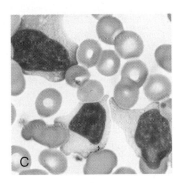

Figure 15–12C   Reactive lymphocytes, cytoplasm indented by adjacent cells

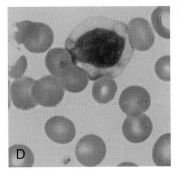

Figure 15–12D   Reactive lymphocyte, radial basophilia

SHAPE: Pleomorphic; easily indented by surrounding cells
SIZE: $10-30\mu$
NUCLEUS: Irregular
    Nucleoli: Occasionally present
    Chromatin: When compared with that of a resting lymphocyte, chromatin pattern is less dense and may be fine and dispersed.
CYTOPLASM: Pale blue to deeply basophilic, may stain unevenly with peripheral or radial basophilia
    Granules: May have increased numbers of azurophilic granules
    Vacuoles: Occasionally
Associated with: Viral infections and other antigenic stimulation, including organ transplantation
NOTE: Although reactive lymphocytes display changes in both nucleus and cytoplasm, they are included in this chapter because the cytoplasmic changes are the more prominent feature.

Table 15–1   MONOCYTE VERSUS REACTIVE LYMPHOCYTE

	Monocyte	Reactive Lymphocyte
Shape	Pleomorphic; may have pseudopodia, which tend to "push away" surrounding cells	Pleomorphic, easily indented by surrounding cells
Size	12–20μ	10–30μ
Nucleus	Round, oval, horseshoe- or kidney-shaped. May have brainlike convolutions.	Irregular, elongated, stretched, occasionally round
Nucleoli	Absent	Occasionally present
Chromatin	Loosely woven, lacy	Variable; clumped to fine and dispersed
Cytoplasm	Blue-gray	Pale blue to deeply basophilic. May stain unevenly.
Granules	Many fine red—may give ground glass appearance	May be a few prominent azurophilic granules
Vacuoles	Absent to numerous	Occasional

Use as many criteria as possible to identify cells. It is often difficult to differentiate cells in isolation; multiple fields should be examined for nuclear and cytoplasmic characteristics. Consider "the company they keep."

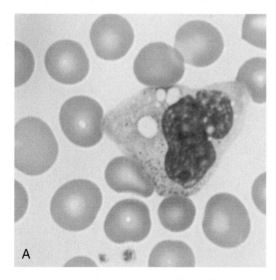

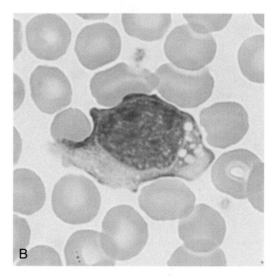

Figure 15–13A   Monocyte. Note the blue-gray cytoplasm with fine red granules. Nucleus has brainlike convolutions. Cell "pushes away" surrounding cells. Vacuoles are present in both of these cells.

Figure 15–13B   Reactive lymphocyte. Note the blue cytoplasm with darker blue periphery. Cell is indented by surrounding cells. Nucleus is elongated. Vacuoles are present in both of these cells.

16

Acute Myeloid Leukemia

ACUTE MYELOID LEUKEMIA, MINIMALLY DIFFERENTIATED
FAB* M0

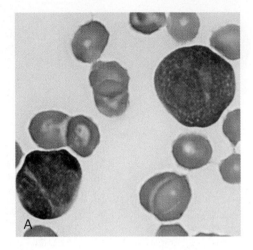

Figure 16–1A   Peripheral blood (×1000)

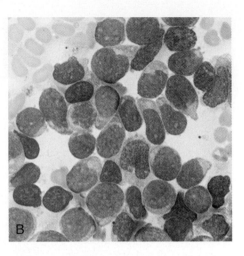

Figure 16–1B   Bone marrow (×500)

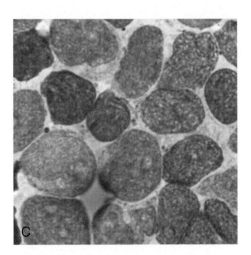

Figure 16–1C   Bone marrow (×1000)

Peripheral Blood: Large agranular blasts, thrombocytopenia

Bone Marrow: >30% blasts all nucleated cells (ANC), >90% blasts nonerythroid cells (NEC), myeloperoxidase (MPO)–negative (see Fig. 21–1A), Sudan Black B (SBB)–negative (see Fig. 21–1B)

*French-American-British classification of acute leukemias

ACUTE MYELOID LEUKEMIA WITHOUT DIFFERENTIATION
FAB M1

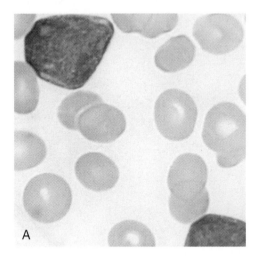

Figure 16–2A   Peripheral blood (×1000)

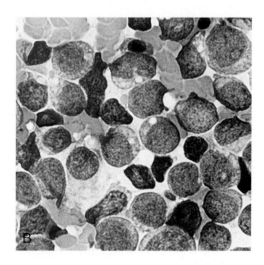

Figure 16–2B   Bone marrow (×500)

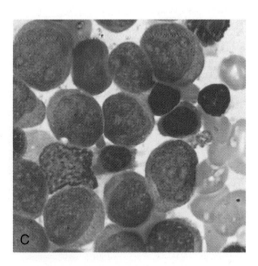

Figure 16–2C   Bone marrow (×1000)

Peripheral Blood: Blasts, thrombocytopenia
Bone Marrow: >30% blasts ANC, >90% blasts NEC, MPO/SBB–positive in ≥3% cells (see Figs. 21–1A and 21–1B)

ACUTE MYELOID LEUKEMIA WITH DIFFERENTIATION
FAB M2

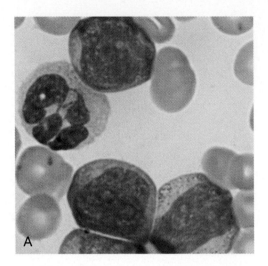

Figure 16–3A   Peripheral blood (×1000)

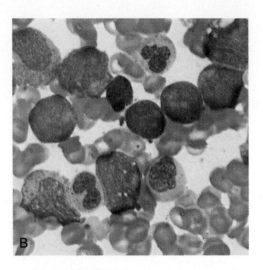

Figure 16–3B   Bone marrow (×500)

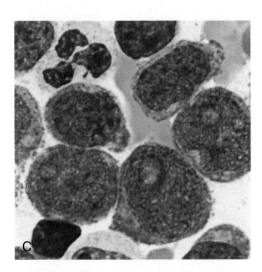

Figure 16–3C   Bone marrow (×1000)

Peripheral Blood: Blasts with some maturation, ±Auer rods, thrombocytopenia
Bone Marrow: >30% blasts ANC, <90% blasts NEC, >10% granulocytic component; <20% monocytic component, maturation beyond promyelocyte stage in >10% of NEC, MPO/SBB–positive in ≥3% cells (see Figs. 21–1A and 21–1B), ±Auer rods

ACUTE PROMYELOCYTIC LEUKEMIA
FAB M3

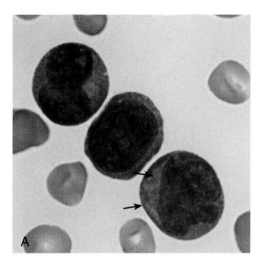

Figure 16–4A   Peripheral blood (×1000)

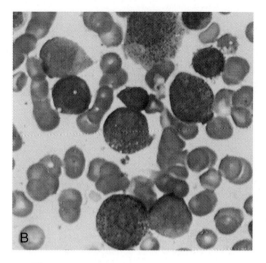

Figure 16–4B   Bone marrow (×500)

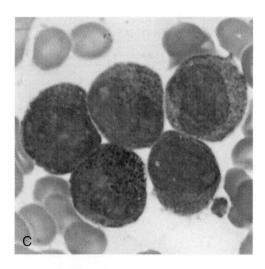

Figure 16–4C   Bone marrow (×1000)

Peripheral Blood: Hypergranular promyelocytes, nuclei often bilobed or kidney-shaped, multiple Auer rods possible, as denoted by arrows in Figure 16–4A

Bone Marrow: Hypergranular promyelocytes, nuclei often bilobed or kidney-shaped, multiple Auer rods; may be in bundles (Faggot cells), MPO/SBB—strongly positive (see Figs. 21–1A and 21–1B)

ACUTE PROMYELOCYTIC LEUKEMIA—MICROGRANULAR VARIANT
FAB M3m

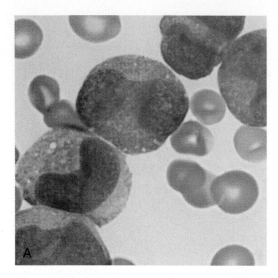

Figure 16–5A   Peripheral blood (×1000)

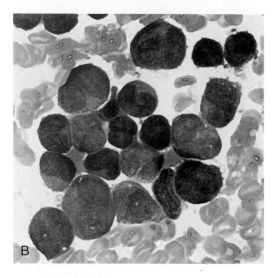

Figure 16–5B   Bone marrow (×500)

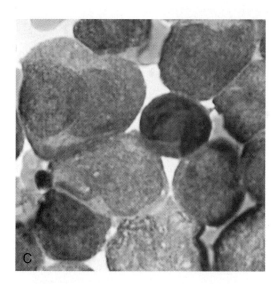

Figure 16–5C   Bone marrow (×1000)

Peripheral Blood: Deeply notched nuclei; granules not visible by light microscopy, but may be
seen on electron microscopy (EM)

Bone Marrow: Agranular promyelocytes, with deeply notched nuclei, MPO/SBB—strongly positive (see Figs. 21–1A and 21–1B)

ACUTE MYELOMONOCYTIC LEUKEMIA
FAB M4

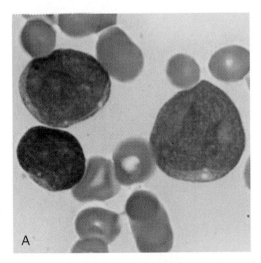

Figure 16–6A Peripheral blood (×1000)

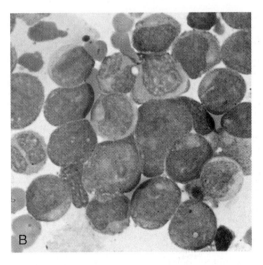

Figure 16–6B Bone marrow (×500)

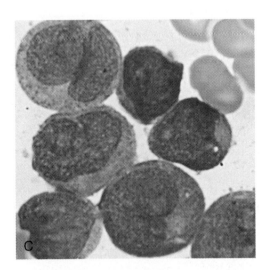

Figure 16–6C Bone marrow (×1000)

Peripheral Blood: Myeloblasts and other immature myeloid cells, monocytoid cells, thrombocy-topenia, ±Auer rods

Bone Marrow: Myeloblasts, promyelocytes, and other myeloid precursors comprise between 30% and 80% NEC, monocytic component >20%, MPO > 3% (see Fig. 21–1A), α-naphthyl butyrate esterase (NBE)–positive (see Fig. 21–1C), ±Auer rods

ACUTE MYELOMONOCYTIC LEUKEMIA WITH EOSINOPHILIA
FAB M4 EO

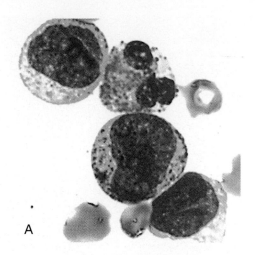

Figure 16–7A   Peripheral blood (×1000)

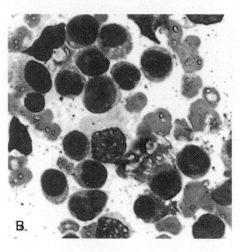

Figure 16–7B   Bone marrow (×500)

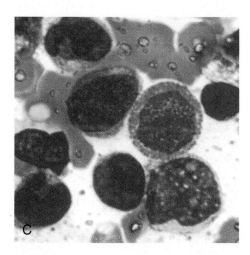

Figure 16–7C   Bone marrow (×1000)

Peripheral Blood: Myeloblasts and other immature myeloid cells, monocytoid cells, thrombocytopenia

Bone Marrow: Myeloblasts, promyelocytes, and other myeloid precursors comprise between 30% and 80% NEC, monocytic component >20%, MPO > 3% (see Fig. 21–1A), NBE-positive (see Fig. 21–1C), ±Auer rods, >5% eosinophils with monocytoid features and basophilic granules

ACUTE MONOCYTIC LEUKEMIA, POORLY DIFFERENTIATED
FAB M5a

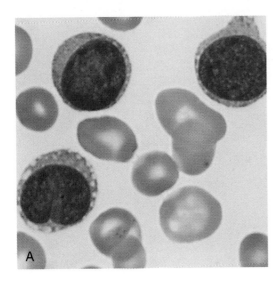

Figure 16–8A   Peripheral blood (×1000)

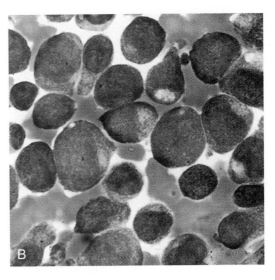

Figure 16–8B   Bone marrow (×500)

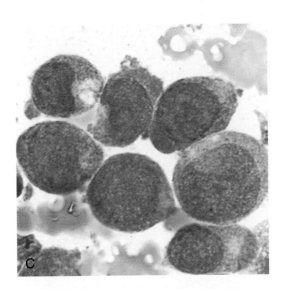

Figure 16–8C   Bone marrow (×1000)

Peripheral Blood: Blasts, thrombocytopenia

Bone Marrow: >30% blasts; >80% have monocytic morphology, granulocytic component <20%, MPO <3% (see Fig. 21–1A), NBE-positive (see Fig. 21–1C)

ACUTE MONOCYTIC LEUKEMIA, WELL-DIFFERENTIATED
FAB M5b

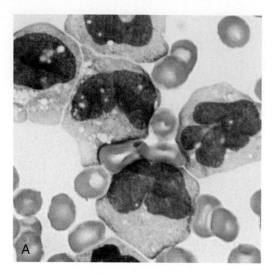

Figure 16–9A   Peripheral blood (×1000)

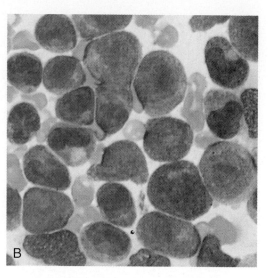

Figure 16–9B   Bone marrow (×500)

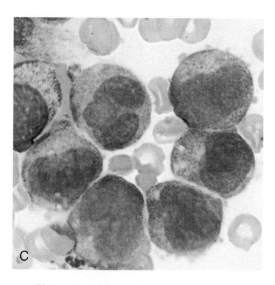

Figure 16–9C   Bone marrow (×1000)

Peripheral Blood: Blasts, monocytoid cells, thrombocytopenia

Bone Marrow: Monocytic component >80%, monoblasts <80% with promonocytes and monocytes, MPO <3% (see Fig. 21–1A), NBE-positive (see Fig. 21–1C)

ACUTE ERYTHROLEUKEMIA
FAB M6

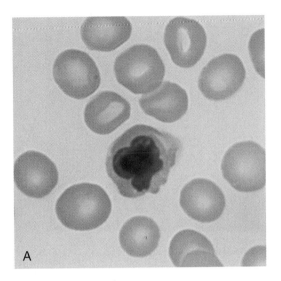

Figure 16–10A   Peripheral blood (×1000)

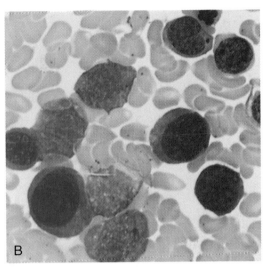

Figure 16–10B   Bone marrow (×500)

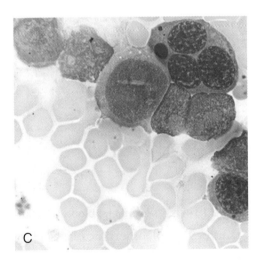

Figure 16–10C   Bone marrow (×1000)

Peripheral Blood: Thrombocytopenia; dimorphic, dichromic erythroid population; basophilic stippling; nucleated erythrocytes; ±blasts

Bone Marrow: ≥30% blasts NEC, ≥50% blasts ANC, bizarre erythroid precursors, periodic acid–Schiff (PAS)–positive with "chunky" or block positivity (see Fig. 21–1D)

ACUTE LYMPHOID LEUKEMIA
FAB* L1

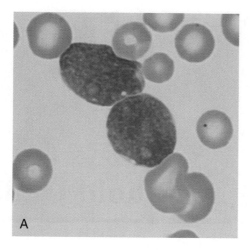

Figure 17–1A Peripheral blood (×1000)

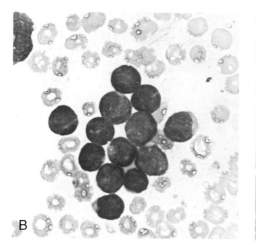

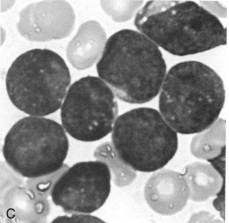

Figure 17–1B Bone marrow (×500)   **Figure 17–1C** Bone marrow (×1000)

Peripheral Blood: ±Blasts, small blasts with scant blue cytoplasm and round nucleoli, thrombocytopenia

Bone Marrow: >30% blasts; homogeneous population, myeloperoxidase (MPO)–negative (see Fig. 21–1A), Sudan Black B (SBB)–negative (see Fig. 21–1B), periodic acid–Schiff (PAS)—variable, often positive (see Fig. 21–1D)

*French-American-British classification of acute leukemia

ACUTE LYMPHOID LEUKEMIA
FAB L2

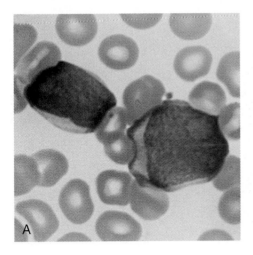

Figure 17–2A   Peripheral blood (×1000)

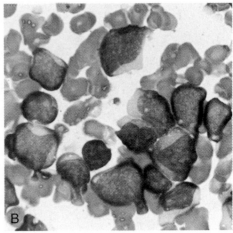

Figure 17–2B   Bone marrow (×500)

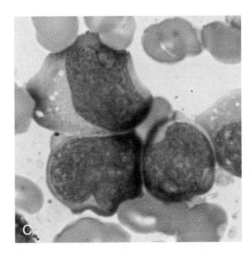

Figure 17–2C   Bone marrow (×1000)

Peripheral Blood: Blasts—2 to 3 times the size of a resting lymphocyte, moderate cytoplasm, irregular nuclear membrane, prominent nucleoli, thrombocytopenia, morphologically difficult to distinguish from acute myeloid leukemia

Bone Marrow: >30% blasts, heterogeneous population, myeloperoxidase (MPO)–negative (see Fig. 21–1A), Sudan Black B (SBB)–negative (see Fig. 21–1B), periodic acid–Schiff (PAS)—variable, often positive (see Fig. 21–1D)

ACUTE LYMPHOID LEUKEMIA
FAB L3

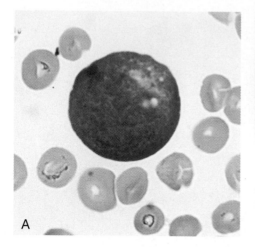

Figure 17–3A   Peripheral blood (×1000)

Figure 17–3B   Bone marrow (×500)

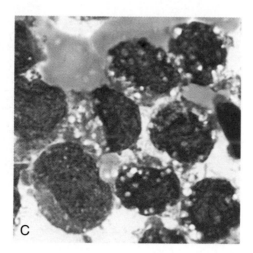

Figure 17–3C   Bone marrow (×1000)

Peripheral Blood: Large blasts with dark blue cytoplasm, vacuoles in cytoplasm, 3–5 nucleoli, thrombocytopenia

Bone Marrow: >30% blasts, homogeneous, myeloperoxidase (MPO)–negative (see Fig. 21–1A), Sudan Black B (SBB)–negative (see Fig. 21–1B), periodic acid–Schiff (PAS)—variable, usually negative (see Fig. 21–1D)

CHAPTER

18

Myeloproliferative Disorders

CHRONIC MYELOID LEUKEMIA (CML)

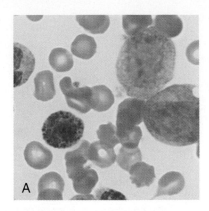

Figure 18–1A   Peripheral blood (×1000)

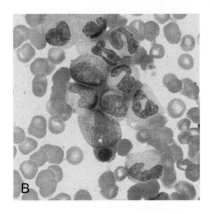

Figure 18–1B   Bone marrow (×500)   **Figure 18–1C**   Bone marrow (×1000)

Peripheral Blood: Marked leukocytosis (usually >50.0 × 10^9/L);
spectrum of myeloid cells with a predominance of myelocytes and
polymorphonuclear neutrophils
myeloblasts and promyelocytes: 1–5%
±pseudo–Pelger-Huët cells
eosinophilia and/or basophilia
monocytosis
Platelets—normal to increased
±Circulating micromegakaryocytes
Leukocyte alkaline phosphatase (LAP)—markedly decreased (see Fig. 21–2)
Bone Marrow: Hypercellular with expansion of granulocyte pool, M:E ratio increased ≥10:1,
myeloblasts and promyelocytes <30%, megakaryocytes—normal to increased;
may be immature and/or atypical

POLYCYTHEMIA VERA (PV)

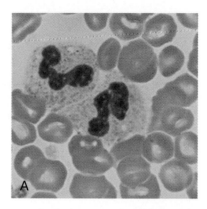

Figure 18–2A   Peripheral blood (×1000)

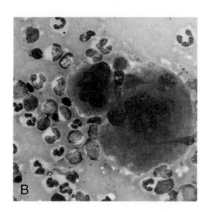

Figure 18–2B   Bone marrow (×500)

Figure 18–2C   Bone marrow (×1000)

Peripheral Blood: Absolute erythrocytosis
  Moderate leukocytosis (12.0–25.0 × 10⁹/L)
      neutrophilia with few metamyelocytes, rare myelocytes
      promyelocytes and myeloblasts extremely rare
      ±eosinophilia and/or basophilia
  Thrombocytosis
  LAP—normal or increased
Bone Marrow: Hypercellular with panhyperplasia, M:E ratio—usually normal, megakaryocytes
  may be abnormal in size and morphology
NOTE: The diagnosis of polycythemia vera is not made on morphology but on the basis of an
  elevated erythrocyte mass and normal oxygen saturation.

ESSENTIAL THROMBOCYTHEMIA (ET)

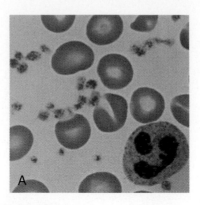

Figure 18–3A   Peripheral blood (×1000)

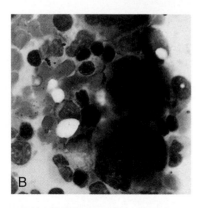

Figure 18–3B   Bone marrow (×500)   **Figure 18–3C**   Bone marrow (×1000)

Peripheral Blood: Marked thrombocytosis ($>600.0 \times 10^9$/L)
abnormal platelet morphology (variations in size, shape, and granulation); often present in clusters

±Leukocytosis: Neutrophilia with bands and metamyelocytes

LAP: Normal or increased (see Fig. 21–2)

Bone Marrow: Hypercellular with expansion of the megakaryocyte pool
large megakaryocytes with abundant cytoplasm may exhibit hyperlobu-
lation

Mild granulocytic hyperplasia
Mild erythrocytic hyperplasia

MYELOFIBROSIS WITH MYELOID METAPLASIA (MMM)
Agnogenic Myeloid Metaplasia (AMM)

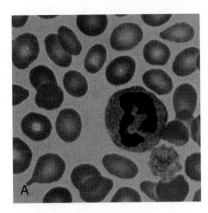

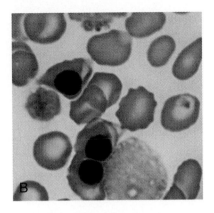

Figure 18–4A Peripheral blood (×1000) (subtle changes)

Figure 18–4B Peripheral blood (×1000) (more advanced case)

Peripheral Blood: Erythrocytes
        dacryocytes common, nucleated erythrocytes, polychromasia
   Leukocytes
      normal, increased, or decreased
      immature granulocytes
      <5% blasts
      ±basophilia and eosinophilia
      morphologic abnormalities
   LAP—normal, increased, or decreased
   Platelets
      low, normal, or increased
      giant bizarre shapes
      abnormal granulation
      ±circulating megakaryocytes

Bone Marrow: Aspiration attempts often result in a dry tap; biopsies exhibit marked fibrosis with islands of hematopoietic activity

CHAPTER 19

Myelodysplastic Syndromes

MYELODYSPLASTIC SYNDROMES

Myelodysplastic syndromes (MDS) are acquired clonal hematologic disorders characterized by progressive cytopenias in peripheral blood, reflecting maturation defects in erythrocytes, leukocytes, and/or platelets.

French-American-British (FAB) Classification of MDS includes
- Refractory anemia (RA)
- Refractory anemia with ringed sideroblasts (RARS)
- Refractory anemia with excess blasts (RAEB)
- Refractory anemia with excess blasts in transformation (RAEB-t)
- Chronic myelomonocytic leukemia (CMML)

Table 19–1 FEATURES OF PERIPHERAL BLOOD AND BONE MARROW IN MYELODYSPLASTIC SYNDROMES (MDS) (FAB CLASSIFICATION)

	Refractory Anemia (RA)	Refractory Anemia with Ringed Siderocytes (RARS)	Refractory Anemia with Excess Blasts (RAEB)	Refractory Anemia with Excess Blasts in Transformation (RAEB-t)	Chronic Myelomonocytic Leukemia (CMML)
% Peripheral blood blasts	<1	<1	<5	≥5	<5
% Bone marrow blasts	<5	<5	5–20	>20, <30	5–20
Other significant findings	<15% RS Oval macrocytes Cytopenias	>15% RS Dimorphic erythrocyte population Oval macrocytes Cytopenias	Oval macrocytes Cytopenias	Absolute monocytosis ($>1.0 \times 10^9$/L) Oval macrocytes	Absolute monocytosis ($>1.0 \times 10^9$/L) Oval macrocytes

RS, ringed sideroblasts.

DYSERYTHROPOIESIS

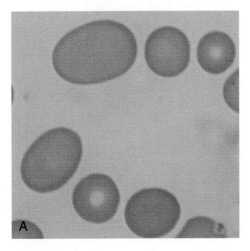

Figure 19–1A   Oval macrocytes (peripheral blood [PB] ×1000)

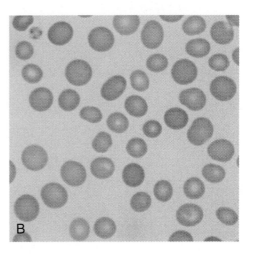

Figure 19–1B   Dimorphic erythrocyte population (PB ×500)

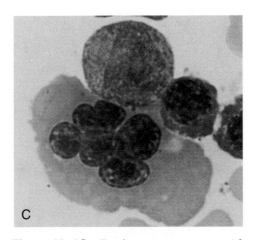

Figure 19–1C   Erythrocyte precursor with multiple nuclei (bone marrow [BM] ×1000)

Evidence of dyserythropoiesis (Figs. 19–1A to 19–1I) may include any or all of the following:
oval macrocytes; hypochromic microcytes; dimorphic erythrocyte population; erythrocyte precursors with >1 nucleus, abnormal nuclear shapes, nuclear bridging, uneven cytoplasmic staining, ringed sideroblasts

NOTE: All figures are ×1000 with Wright-Giemsa stain, unless otherwise noted.

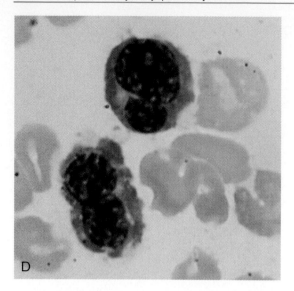

Figure 19–1D Erythrocyte precursor with abnormal nuclear shape, bilobed (BM ×1000)

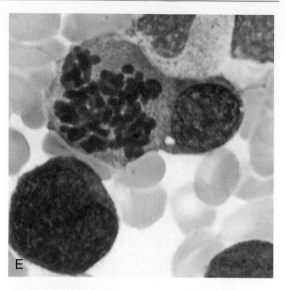

Figure 19–1E Erythrocyte precursor with abnormal nuclear shape (bilobed, with one nucleus in mitosis, demonstrating asynchrony) (BM ×1000)

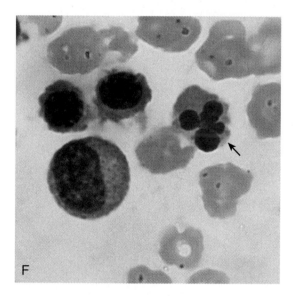

Figure 19–1F Erythrocyte precursor with abnormal nuclear shape (BM ×1000)

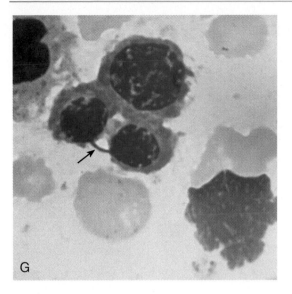

Figure 19–1G   Erythrocyte precursor with nuclear bridging (BM ×1000)

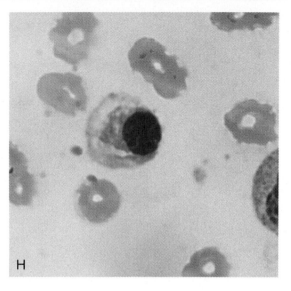

Figure 19–1H   Erythrocyte precursor with uneven cytoplasmic staining (BM ×1000)

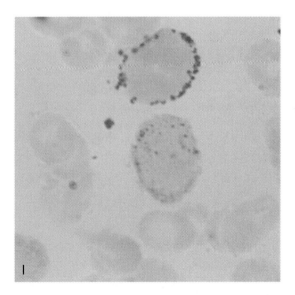

Figure 19–1I   Ringed sideroblast (iron stain, BM ×1000)

DYSMYELOPOIESIS

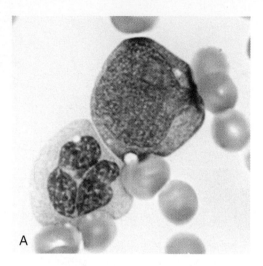

Figure 19–2A   Abnormal granulation, agranular polymorphonuclear neutrophil

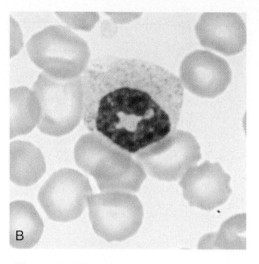

Figure 19–2B   Abnormal nuclear shapes, neutrophil with circular (donut) nucleus

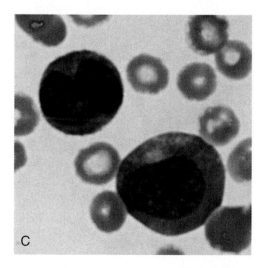

Figure 19–2C   Persistent basophilic cytoplasm

Evidence of dysmyelopoiesis (Figs. 19–2A to 19–2E) may include any or all of the following: abnormal granulation, abnormal nuclear shapes, persistent basophilic cytoplasm, uneven cytoplasmic staining

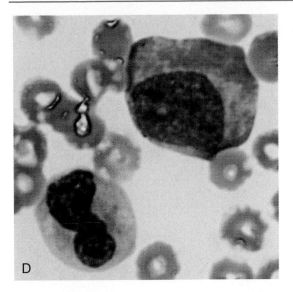

Figure 19–2D   Uneven cytoplasmic staining

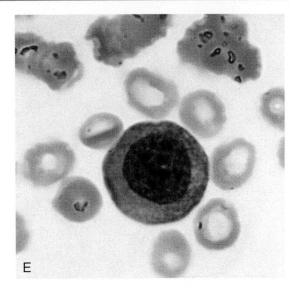

Figure 19–2E   Uneven cytoplasmic staining

DYSMEGAKARYOPOIESIS

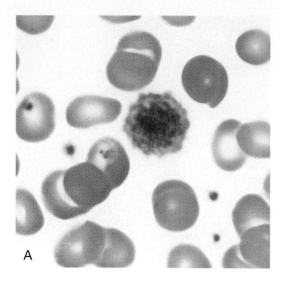

Figure 19–3A   Giant platelet

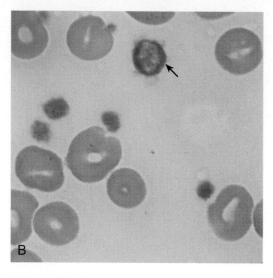

Figure 19–3B   Platelet with abnormal granulation

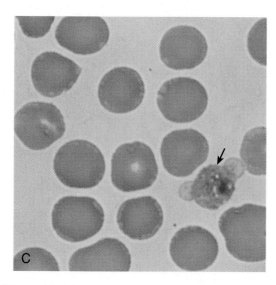

Figure 19–3C   Platelet with abnormal granulation

Evidence of dysmegakaryopoiesis (Figs. 19–3A to 19–3G) may include any or all of the following: giant platelets, platelets with abnormal granulation, circulating micromegakaryocytes, large mononuclear megakaryocytes, abnormal nuclear shapes

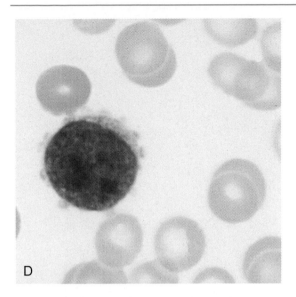

Figure 19–3D   Circulating micromegakaryocyte (PB ×1000)

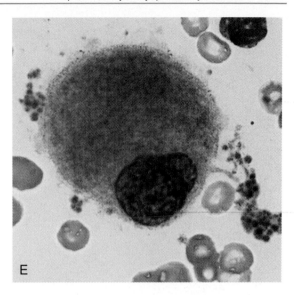

Figure 19–3E   Large mononuclear megakaryocyte (BM ×1000)

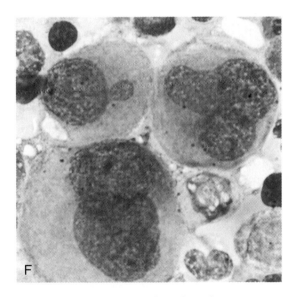

Figure 19–3F   Abnormal nuclear shape, uneven nuclei (BM ×1000)

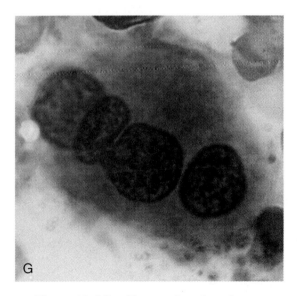

Figure 19–3G   Abnormal nuclear shapes, separate nuclei (BM ×1000)

20

Malignant Lymphoproliferative Disorders

Malignant lymphoproliferative disorders frequently are derived from a single clone of cells. Although this group of diseases involves lymphocytes, the morphologic presentation is variable. The integration of clinical and morphologic disease features with immunophenotyping and cytogenetic and molecular studies is necessary for appropriate recognition and classification. Only representative samples are included in this atlas.

NOTE: Any absolute lymphocytosis in an adult should be investigated.

PROLYMPHOCYTIC LEUKEMIA (PLL)

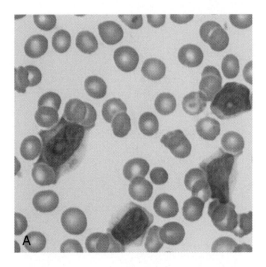

Figure 20–1A   Peripheral blood (PB ×500)

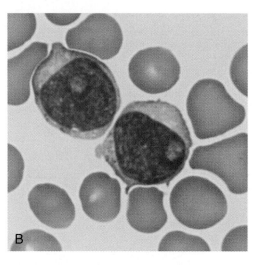

Figure 20–1B   (PB ×1000)

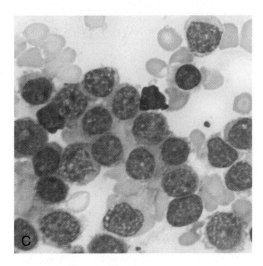

Figure 20–1C   Bone marrow (BM ×500)

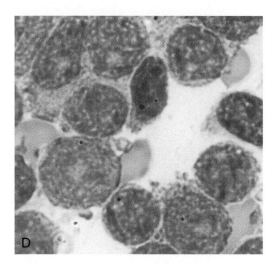

Figure 20–1D   (BM ×1000)

Peripheral Blood: Absolute lymphocytosis, usually >100.0 × 10^9/L, relatively large cells having one prominent nucleolus, chromatin structure intermediate between that of a blast and a mature lymphocyte, relatively uniform within a given patient, anemia, thrombocytopenia

Bone Marrow: Predominantly prolymphocytes with very few residual hematopoietic cells

CHRONIC LYMPHOCYTIC LEUKEMIA (CLL)

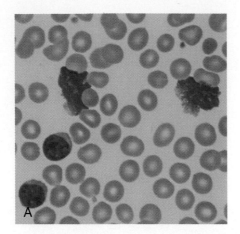

Figure 20–2A   (PB ×500)

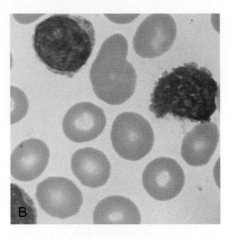

Figure 20–2B   (PB ×1000)

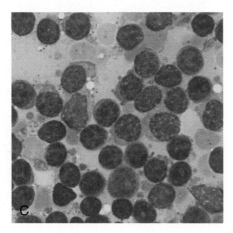

Figure 20–2C   (BM ×500)

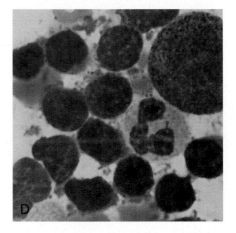

Figure 20–2D   (BM ×1000)

Peripheral Blood: Absolute sustained lymphocytosis ($10\text{–}150 \times 10^9/\text{L}$), homogeneous appearance within a given patient, mature-appearing lymphocytes with round nuclei and block type chromatin, cytoplasm scant or moderate, lymphocytes more fragile than normal, leading to "smudge" cells
normocytic normochromic anemia, which increases with disease progression, approximately 10% develop a hemolytic anemia
thrombocytopenia develops with disease progression

Bone Marrow: ≥30% lymphocytes

HAIRY CELL LEUKEMIA (HCL)

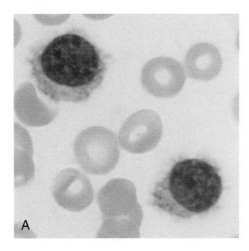

Figure 20–3A   (PB ×1000)

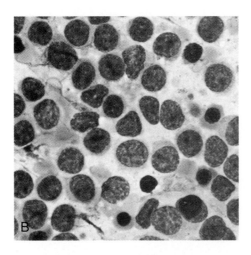

Figure 20–3B   (BM ×500)

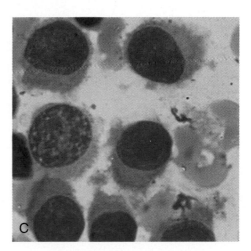

Figure 20–3C   (BM ×1000)

Peripheral Blood: Pancytopenia, reniform to oval nuclei with diffuse homogeneous chromatin, may have a single nucleolus, cytoplasm irregular and gray-blue with delicate hairlike cytoplasmic projections

Bone Marrow: Aspirate difficult to obtain due to marrow fibrosis (dry tap), cells more easily distinguished by phase or electron microscopy, cells positive by the tartrate-resistant acid phosphatase (TRAP) stain (see Figure 21–2)

WALDENSTRÖM'S MACROGLOBULINEMIA

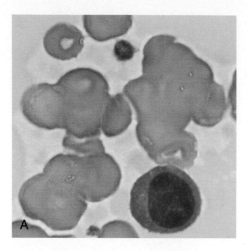

Figure 20–4A (PB ×1000)

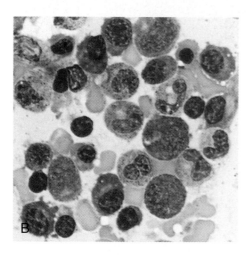

Figure 20–4B (BM ×500)

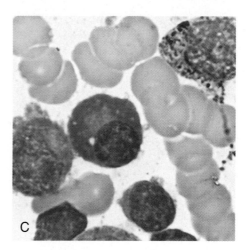

Figure 20–4C (BM ×1000)

Peripheral Blood: Leukocyte count usually normal, rare plasmacytoid cell or plasma cell, normocytic normochromic anemia with rouleaux, normal to decreased platelet numbers, excess protein may cause a blue precipitate, as demonstrated in Figure 20–4A

Bone Marrow: Hypercellular with plasmacytoid infiltrates

NOTE: This disease may be distinguished from multiple myeloma and heavy chain disease by immunoelectrophoresis.

MULTIPLE MYELOMA

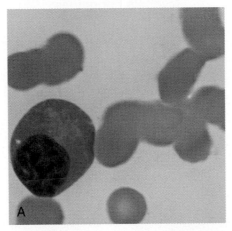

Figure 20–5A (PB ×1000)

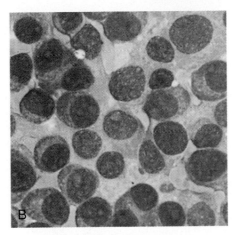

Figure 20–5B (BM ×500)

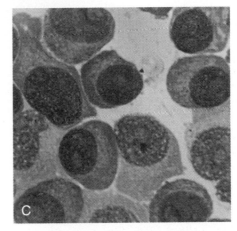

Figure 20–5C (BM ×1000)

Peripheral Blood: Possible neutropenia, rare abnormal circulating plasma cell, normocytic normochromic anemia, rouleaux, platelet count normal to decreased. If greater
than 2.0×10^9/L plasma cells are circulating in the peripheral blood, plasma
cell leukemia is present.

NOTE: The background of Wright-stained blood smears may be blue owing to abnormal
amounts of immunoglobulin.

Bone Marrow: >10% abnormal plasma cells; often >30%, larger than normal plasma cell with
increased N/C ratio, immature in appearance, abnormal nuclear chromatin,
±nucleoli, nucleus may be centrally located, ±multinucleated, possible loss of
nuclear hof, cytoplasm may be pale blue or dark, cytoplasm may contain immunoglobulin inclusions

NOTE: This disease may be distinguished from Waldenström's macroglobulinemia and heavy
chain disease by immunoelectrophoresis.

SÉZARY SYNDROME
Mycosis Fungoides

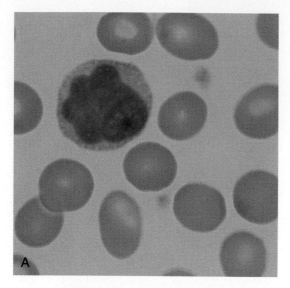 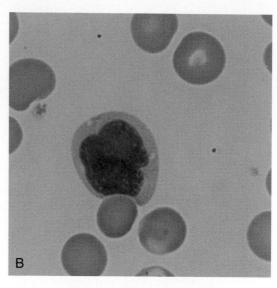

Figure 20–6A (PB ×1000)   **Figure 20–6B** (PB ×1000)

Peripheral Blood: 15–25μ, cerebriform nucleus with coarse chromatin and inconspicuous
              nucleoli
          NOTE: Sézary cells in the peripheral blood are morphologically altered T
              cells and represent the cutaneous T-cell lymphoma, mycosis fun-
              goides, which involves the skin.
          PAS positive—see Figure 21–1D.
Bone Marrow: NA

NON-HODGKIN LYMPHOMAS

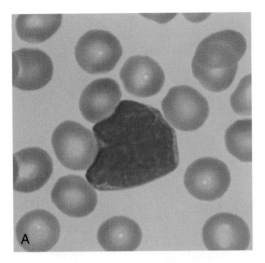

Figure 20–7A (PB ×1000)

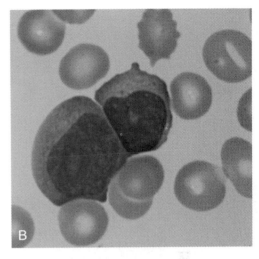

Figure 20–7B (PB ×1000)

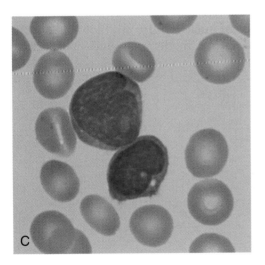

Figure 20–7C (PB ×1000)

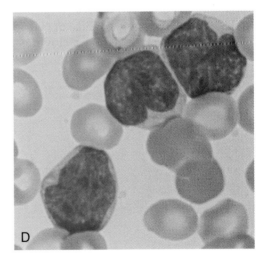

Figure 20–7D (PB ×1000)

Peripheral Blood: A variety of lymphoma cells has been illustrated because occasionally lymphoma cells are found in the peripheral blood. The diagnosis of lymphoma is determined by lymph node biopsy, immunophenotyping, and cytogenetics.

Bone Marrow: NA

Figure 21–1 demonstrates stains that are used primarily to differentiate acute leukemias. Results are summarized in Table 21–1.

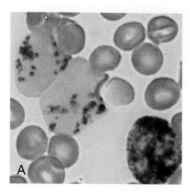

A

Figure 21–1A Myeloperoxidase (MPX) (Bone marrow [BM], ×1000)

Stains granules containing peroxidase, that is, primary granules in neutrophils and granules in eosinophils and monocytes.

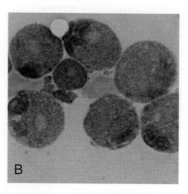

B

Figure 21–1B Sudan Black B (SBB) (BM ×1000)

Stains lipids, including neutral fat, phospholipids, and sterols. Parallels myeloperoxidase reaction.

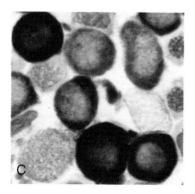

C

Figure 21–1C α-Naphthyl butyrate esterase (NBE) (BM ×1000)

Esterase hydrolyzes an ester. Diffusely positive in monocytes and negative or focally positive in the neutrophil series.

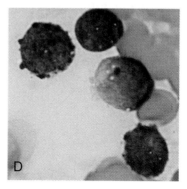

D

Figure 21–1D Periodic acid–Schiff (PAS) (BM ×1000)

Stains carbohydrates, primarily glycogen. Block positivity is associated with acute lymphoblastic leukemia and early precursors of FAB M-6 leukemia. Later precursors show diffuse positivity.

Table 21–1 SIMPLIFIED ACUTE LEUKEMIA REACTION CHART

Condition	Myeloperoxidase	Sudan Black B	α-Naphthyl Butyrate Esterase (NBE)	PAS
ALL (L1–3)	–	–	–	Varied; usually positive in L1 & L2
AML (M1–3)	+	+	–	Varied
AMML (M-4)	+	+	+	Varied
AMOL (M-5)	–	±	+	Varied
Erythroid (M-6)	–	–	–	Positive in erythrocyte precursors

PAS, periodic acid–Schiff stain; ALL, acute lymphoblastic leukemia; AML, acute myelogenous leukemia; AMML, acute myelomonocytic leukemia; AMOL, acute monocytic leukemia.
From Rodak B: Diagnostic Hematology. Philadelphia, WB Saunders, 1995.

TARTRATE-RESISTANT LEUKOCYTE ACID PHOSPHATASE (TRAP)

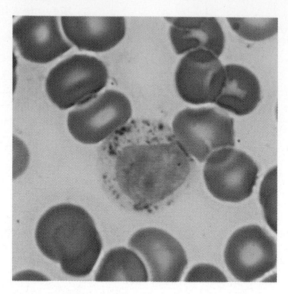

Figure 21–2   Tartrate-resistant leukocyte acid phosphatase (TRAP)

Positive in most cases of hairy cell leukemia. Those cells contain acid phosphatase and remain positive after the addition of L(+)-tartaric acid.

LEUKOCYTE ALKALINE PHOSPHATASE (LAP)

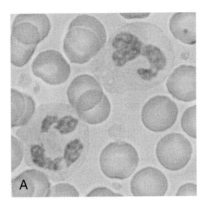

Figure 21–3A Leukocyte alkaline phosphatase (LAP)–negative reaction (0) (PB ×1000)

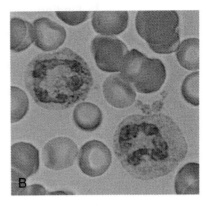

Figure 21–3B LAP (1+) (PB ×1000)

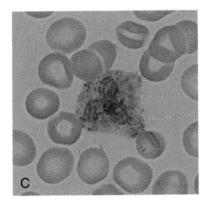

Figure 21–3C LAP (2+) (PB ×1000)

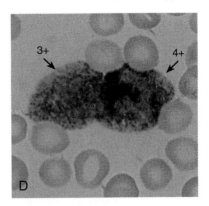

Figure 21–3D LAP (3+, 4+) (PB ×1000)

LAP is an enzyme found in secondary granules of neutrophils. LAP activity is scored from 0 to 4+ in the mature polymorphonuclear neutrophils and bands. One hundred cells are scored and added together for the LAP score. A normal score is approximately 20 to 100. Low (<20) scores may be found in untreated chronic myeloid leukemia, paroxysmal nocturnal hemoglobinuria, sideroblastic anemia, and myelodysplastic syndromes. Higher scores may be found in leukemoid reactions, polycythemia vera, and the third trimester of pregnancy. See Table 21–2.

PLASMODIUM SPECIES

The following are representative examples of the developmental stages of malaria that can be seen in the peripheral blood. Detailed criteria for identification of species may be found in a parasitology text.

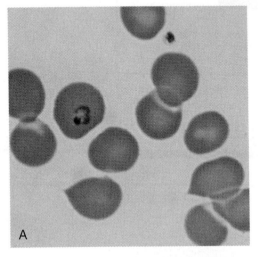

Figure 22–1A *Plasmodium* species (peripheral blood [PB] ×1000)

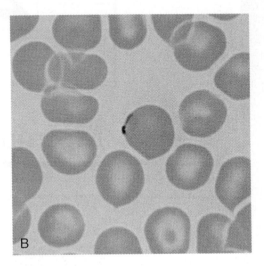

Figure 22–1B Appliqué form (PB ×1000)

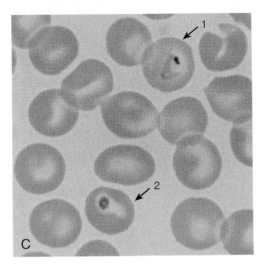

Figure 22–1C Platelet versus malaria: 1- malaria 2- platelet (PB ×1000)

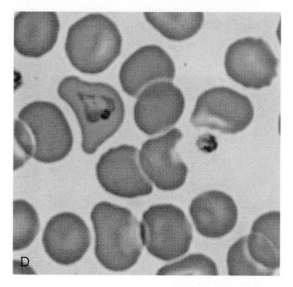

Figure 22–1D *Plasmodium* species (PB ×1000)

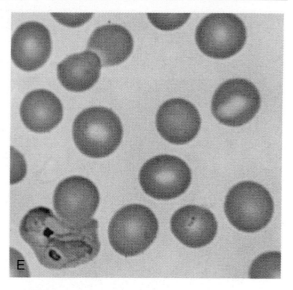

Figure 22–1E *Plasmodium* species (PB ×1000)

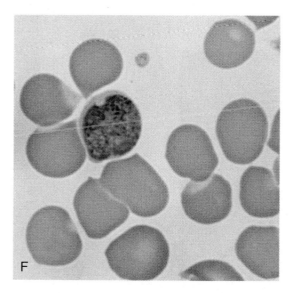

Figure 22–1F *Plasmodium* species (PB ×1000)

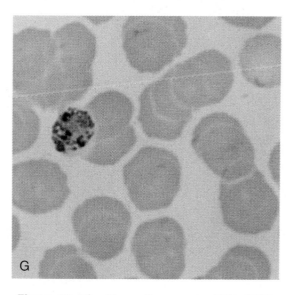

Figure 22–1G *Plasmodium* species (PB ×1000)

BABESIA

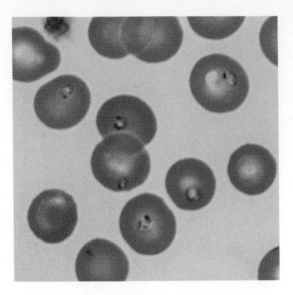

Figure 22–2 *Babesia microti* (PB ×1000)

Babesia species may be confused morphologically with *Plasmodium falciparum* but lack of pigment, and absence of life cycle stages help differentiate *Babesia* from *P. falciparum*. Another differentiating factor is the presence of extracellular organisms that may be seen in *Babesia* but not in *P. falciparum*.

LOA LOA

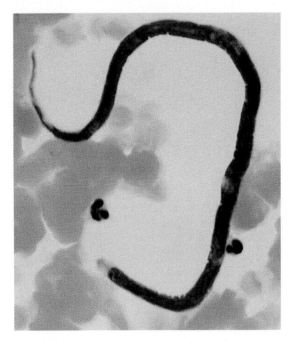

Figure 22–3 Loa Loa, a microfilaria (PB original magnification ×1000)

Loa loa, a microfilaria. Other microfilariae rarely may be seen in the peripheral blood.

TRYPANOSOMES

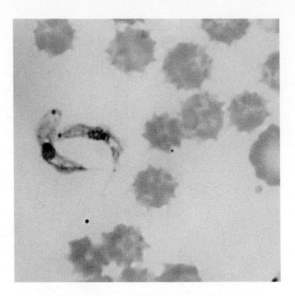

Figure 22–4   Trypanosomes (PB ×1000)

Trypanosomes, an example of hemoflagellates that may occasionally be encountered in the peripheral blood.

FUNGI

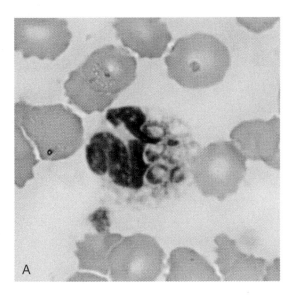

Figure 22–5A   *Histoplasma capsulatum* (PB ×1000)

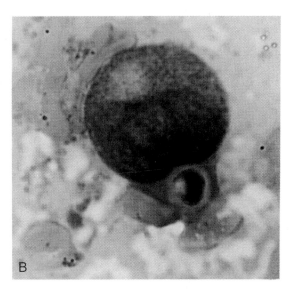

Figure 22–5B   *Cryptococcus neoformans* (bone marrow ×1000)

CELLS OCCASIONALLY SEEN IN BONE MARROW
Fat Cell

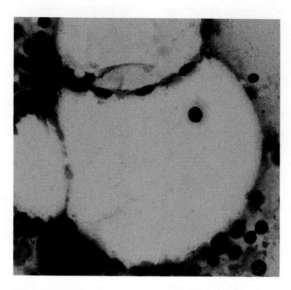

Figure 23–1 Fat cell (bone marrow [BM] ×500)

Description: large round cell, 50–80μ; cytoplasm filled with one or several large fat vacuoles colorless to pale blue; nucleus small, round to oval, and eccentric; chromatin coarse; nucleoli seldom seen

Mitosis

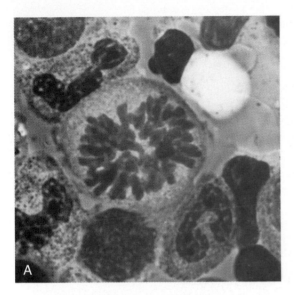

Figure 23–2A   Mitosis (BM ×1000)

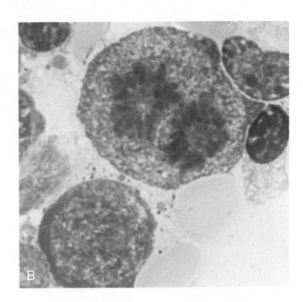

Figure 23–2B   Mitosis (BM ×1000)

Mitotic figure—a cell that is dividing

Erythroblastic Island

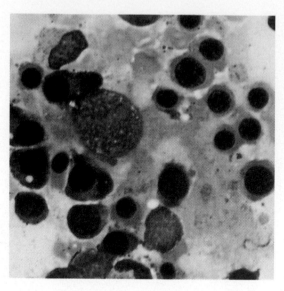

Figure 23–3   Erythroblastic island (nurse cell) (BM ×500)

Iron-laden macrophage surrounded by developing erythroblasts

Bone Cells

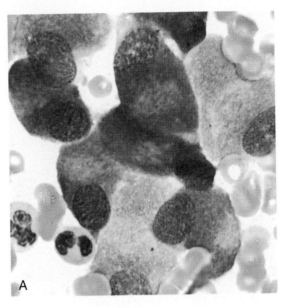

Figure 23–4A Osteoblasts (BM original magnification ×1000)

SIZE: 30µ
Appearance: Comet or tadpole shaped. Single round eccentrically placed nucleus, may be partially extruded. Abundant cytoplasm with chromophobic area located away from nucleus. Often appear in groups. Function in synthesis of bone.

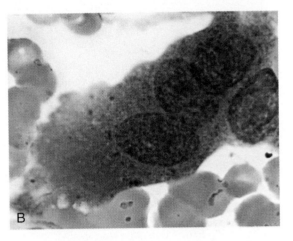

Figure 23–4B Osteoclast (BM original magnification ×1000)

SIZE: Very large, greater than 100µ
Appearance: Cell is irregularly shaped with a ruffled border. Multinucleated; nuclei are round to oval, separate and distinct, and show very little variation in nuclear size. Nucleoli usually visible. Cytoplasm may vary from slightly basophilic to very acid-ophilic. Coarse granules may be present. Osteoclasts function in the resorption of bone.

Metastatic Tumor Cells

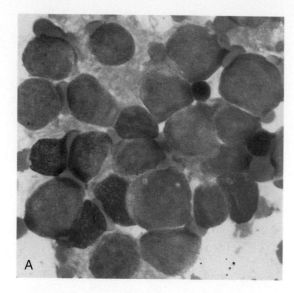

Figure 23–5A Metastatic tumor (BM ×500)   **Figure 23–5B**   Metastatic tumor (BM ×1000)

Cells are variable in size and shape within the same tumor clump. Nuclei vary in size and staining characteristics. Nucleoli are usually visible. It is difficult to distinguish one cell from another due to "molding" of cells.

Endothelial Cells

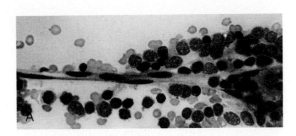

Figure 23–6A Endothelial cells (BM original magnification ×500)

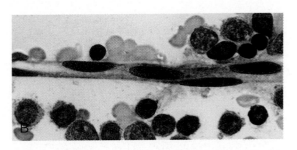

Figure 23–6B Endothelial cells (BM original magnification ×1000)

Large elongated cells, 20–30μ. One oval nucleus with dense chromatin; nucleoli not visible. Function is to line blood vessels.

Plasma Cell Variations

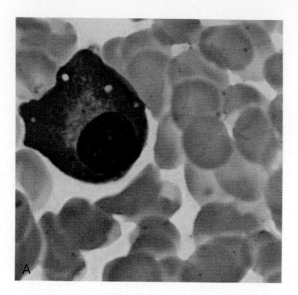

Figure 23–7A   Flame cell (BM ×1000)

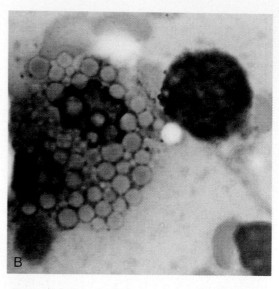

Figure 23–7B   Mott cell, grape cell, morula cell (BM ×1000)

Plasma cell with red cytoplasm due to high concentration of glycoprotein

Plasma cell containing multiple round globules of immunoglobulin, which stain pink, colorless, or blue

ERYTHROCYTE ARTIFACTS

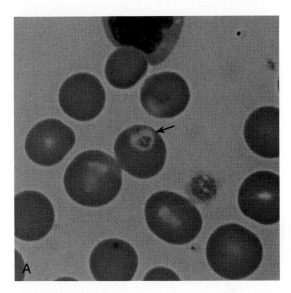

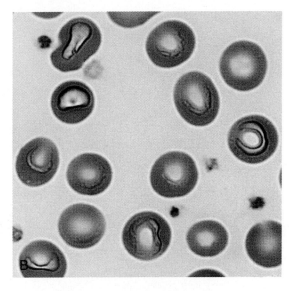

Figure 23–8A   Platelet on RBC, may be confused with malarial parasite (peripheral blood [PB] ×1000)

Figure 23–8B   Water artifact, may be confused with malaria or Cabot ring (PB ×1000)

LEUKOCYTE ARTIFACT

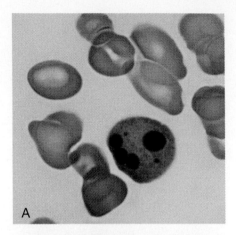

Figure 23–9A   Pyknosis (PB ×1000)

Description: Nuclear degeneration appearing as a darkly stained structure with less mass

Associated with: Peripheral smears made from old blood; cell death

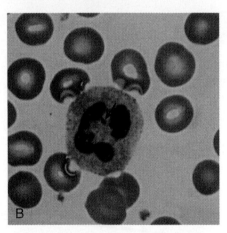

Figure 23–9B   Barr body (PB ×1000)

Description: Small, round, well-defined projection of nuclear chromatin connected to the nucleus by a strand of chromatin

Significance: None

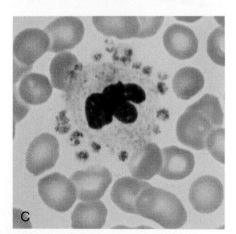

Figure 23–9C   Platelet satellitism (PB ×1000)

Description: Platelets adhering to neutrophils

Associated with: Blood collected in EDTA in rare individuals; may cause falsely decreased platelet counts

Index

Note: Page numbers followed by t refer to tables.